Bone Tumor Imaging

Xiaoguang Cheng · Yongbin Su
Mingqian Huang

Bone Tumor Imaging

Case Studies in Hip and Knee

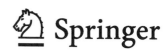

中国协和医科大学出版社
Peking Union Medical College Press

Springer

Xiaoguang Cheng
Department of Radiology
Beijing Jishuitan Hospital
Beijing
China

Yongbin Su
Department of Radiology
Beijing Jishuitan Hospital
Beijing
China

Mingqian Huang
Department of Radiology, Renaissance
School of Medicine
Stony Brook University Hospital
Stony Brook, NY
USA

ISBN 978-981-13-9929-9   ISBN 978-981-13-9927-5   (eBook)
https://doi.org/10.1007/978-981-13-9927-5

This Springer imprint is published by the registered company Springer Nature Singapore Pte Ltd. The registered company address is: 152 Beach Road, #21-01/04 Gateway East, Singapore 189721, Singapore

Foreword

Beijing Jishuitan Hospital has a long history and experience in the diagnosis and treatment of various orthopedic diseases. Despite this abundant experience, the diagnosis of bone tumors remains difficult because of the low morbidity of this condition. Professor Song Xianwen, known as the father of Chinese bone tumors, recalls the establishment of the Chinese bone tumor treatment team in the 1970s and said that "After we had done a lot of clinical work and treated hundreds of orthopaedic patients, we found the complexity of bone tumors… the diagnosing of bone tumors needed the combination of clinical, radiological test and pathological result…." The diagnosis of bone tumors is difficult because bone tumors are a type of orthopedic disease and so have common imaging features with other orthopedic diseases such as congenital abnormalities and degenerative bone disease. Furthermore, there are similarities between bone tumors and metabolic bone disease, and even between the different subtypes of bone tumors.

The World Health Organization's classification system for bone tumors has undergone a transition from being based on histoembryology to histogenesis. The introduction of bone tumor "radiomics" has also further revealed the complexity of bone tumors. The complexity of bone tumors necessitates a combination of clinical, radiological, and pathological findings for accurate diagnosis.

One point that requires special emphasis is that even though some people think that pathological diagnosis is the "gold standard" in combination diagnosis, imaging is actually more reliable than pathology for diagnosing some types of bone tumors. Therefore, in general, we believe that imaging should be the basis for the final diagnosis of bone tumors.

The study of bone tumors requires strong integration of theories and practice. These theories are only fully assimilated after continuous practice. Thus, the importance of practice is endorsed by many famous professors in Beijing Jishuitan Hospital. Professor Song Xianwen from the Department of Bone Tumors and Professor Wang Yunzhao have done a lot of work in determining the correlations between histology and radiology.

I recall Professor Wang Yunzhao holding an imaging meeting in a small room that was about 6 m^2; this meeting was so popular that most of the doctors had to listen from outside the room. This tradition of discussing imaging and the thirst for practical knowledge drive us all. The good news is that this tradition has been inherited by the Department of Radiology in Beijing Jishuitan Hospital. The writing of this book is the cumulative product of continuous practice and imaging meetings that have been held over the past several decades.

This book contains high-quality images, which will increase the ability of clinicians to use imaging to diagnose bone tumors. I believe that there are at least two important benefits to be gained from this book. The first one is the provision of examples of typical radiological findings of bone tumors, which can be consulted as needed. The second one is the description of the analysis process used in bone tumor imaging diagnosis. This describes a real practice that can help the reader to train, verify, and improve his or her diagnostic skills and finally become a "master of bone tumor imaging diagnosis."

In conclusion, this book is a crystallization of collective wisdom that contains rich content and detailed information that is both scientific and practical. This book provides doctors and students with a valuable reference related to bone tumors, which is important in increasing the ability of clinicians to use imaging to diagnose bone tumors.

I am pleased to write the foreword for this book and hope that its publication aids in the development of bone tumor radiology in China.

June 20, 2018   Niu Xiaohui
Department of Orthopaedic Oncology Surgery
Beijing Jishuitan Hospital
Beijing, China

Preface

The correct diagnosis of bone tumor and tumor-like lesions is challenging due to the low prevalence, lack of features, and the variety of bone tumors. The close teamwork of orthopedist, radiologist, and pathologist is the key to meeting this challenge.

The Bone Tumor Department of Beijing Jishuitan Hospital, founded in 1984, was the first center to specialize in bone tumor treatment in China and is well regarded both in China and abroad. Professor Wang Yunzhao, the most famous musculoskeletal radiologist in China, established the Department of Radiology and performed extensive radiology-pathology correlation studies on bone tumors. He was very good at the diagnosis of bone tumors and accumulated a rich database of case studies. Fellows from all over China participated in the bone tumor training course in the department every year. However, we found a lack of books about bone tumors, particularly books with a case-based approach. Therefore, a few years ago we started to collect this series of bone tumors, with carefully selected cases that included comprehensive X-ray, CT, and MRI studies. We present the cases as in the way of the morning roundtable discussion at Jishuitan Hospital, pointing out the key features of each case.

One of the features of this book is that we document the real roundtable discussion of cases in our department. Usually, a young radiologist presents the case with medical history, then the residents or fellows read the images and propose possible differential diagnosis, followed by the attending radiologist, pros and cons of the opinion of the residents, then the two most experienced professors, Cheng Xiaoguang and Gu Xiang, present their opinion on the case. Finally, the pathological finding is presented and carefully correlated with the radiological findings, to find the pros and cons of the diagnosis. In some cases, if the pathological finding was inconsistent with radiology or orthopedics, then the case was sent to the pathology department with a request for a review. Finally, the treatment and follow-up of the patients by the orthopedist is an important part of the discussion. This book exemplifies the close teamwork required between radiologists, orthopedists, and pathologists.

   We greatly appreciate the hard work of graduates and fellows in sorting out the cases and documentation. The publication of this first edition of *Bone Tumor Imaging: Case Studies in Hip and Knee* would not have been possible without the help of the Peking Union Medical College Press, and Lei Nan in particular.

Beijing, China   Xiaoguang Cheng
Stony Brook, NY, USA   Mingqian Huang
Beijing, China   Yongbin Su
July 6, 2019

Contents

Authors and Collaborators

Authors

Xiaoguang Cheng, MD Department of Radiology, Beijing Jishuitan Hospital, Beijing, People's Republic of China

Health Science Center, Peking University, Beijing, People's Republic of China

Yongbin Su, MD Department of Radiology, Beijing Jishuitan Hospital, Beijing, People's Republic of China

Mingqian Huang, MD Department of Radiology, Renaissance School of Medicine, Stony Brook University Hospital, Stony Brook, NY, USA

List of Collaborators

Wei Cai Department of Radiology, Beijing Jishuitan Hospital, Beijing, People's Republic of China

Jia Chen Department of Radiology, Guizhou Orthopedics Hospital, Guiyang, Guizhou, People's Republic of China

Qi-Chun Chen Department of Radiology, The Second Hospital of Anhui Medical University, Hefei, Anhui, People's Republic of China

Xiang-Shu Chen Department of Radiology, Beijing Jishuitan Hospital, Beijing, People's Republic of China

Yi Ding Department of Pathology, Beijing Jishuitan Hospital, Beijing, People's Republic of China

Kang-Chen Gu Department of Radiology, The Second Hospital of Anhui Medical University, Hefei, Anhui, People's Republic of China

Xiang Gu Department of Radiology, Beijing Jishuitan Hospital, Beijing, People's Republic of China

Song Guan Department of Radiology, The Second Hospital of Anhui Medical University, Hefei, Anhui, People's Republic of China

Zhe Guo, MD Department of Radiology, Beijing Jishuitan Hospital, Beijing, People's Republic of China

Ze-Pu Hao Department of Radiology, Cangzhou Hospital of Integrated TCM-WM, Canzhou, Hebei, People's Republic of China

Wen Jiang Department of Radiology, Beijing Jishuitan Hospital, Beijing, People's Republic of China

Kai Li, PhD Department of Radiology, Beijing Jishuitan Hospital, Beijing, People's Republic of China

Xin-Min Li Department of Radiology, Beijing Jishuitan Hospital, Beijing, People's Republic of China

Xin-Tong Li Department of Radiology, Beijing Jishuitan Hospital, Beijing, People's Republic of China

Yi-Xuan Li Department of Radiology, Huailai County Hospital, Huailai, Hebei, People's Republic of China

Ning Liu Department of Radiology, Bethune Memorial Hospital of Tang County, Tang, Hebei, People's Republic of China

Yan-Dong Liu Department of Radiology, Beijing Jishuitan Hospital, Beijing, People's Republic of China

Lu-Xin Lou Department of Radiology, Beijing Jishuitan Hospital, Beijing, People's Republic of China

Xiao-Lan Luo Department of Radiology, People's Hospital of Deyang City, Deyang, Sichuan, People's Republic of China

Yi-Min Ma, MD Department of Radiology, Beijing Jishuitan Hospital, Beijing, People's Republic of China

Wen Song Department of Radiology, Kangji Hospital, Renqiu, Hebei, People's Republic of China

Jia-Nan Tao Department of Medical Imaging, Beijing Huairou Hospital, Huairou, Beijing, People's Republic of China

Chen Wang Department of Radiology, Beijing Jishuitan Hospital, Beijing, People's Republic of China

Sheng-Yang Wang Department of Medical Imaging, Xuzhou Renci Hospital, Xuzhou, Jiangsu, People's Republic of China

Tao Wang, MD Department of Orthopaedic Oncology, Beijing Jishuitan Hospital, Beijing, People's Republic of China

Xin-Guang Wang Department of Radiology, Xingtai Third Hospital, Xingtai, Hebei, People's Republic of China

Shu-Lian Xia Department of Radiology, Fifth Hospital in Wuhan, Wuhan, Hubei, People's Republic of China

Guang-You Xie Department of Radiology, Guizhou Provincial People's Hospital, Guiyang, Guizhou, People's Republic of China

Li Xu Department of Radiology, Beijing Jishuitan Hospital, Beijing, People's Republic of China

Xiao-Ming Xu Department of Radiology, Beijing Jishuitan Hospital, Beijing, People's Republic of China

Dong Yan Department of Radiology, Beijing Jishuitan Hospital, Beijing, People's Republic of China

Jun Yang Department of Radiology, The First Hospital of Fangshan District, Beijing, People's Republic of China

Ruo-Pei Yang Department of Radiology, Beijing Jishuitan Hospital, Beijing, People's Republic of China

Wen-Jun Yao Department of Radiology, The Second Hospital of Anhui Medical University, Hefei, Anhui, People's Republic of China

Yan-Ni Zeng Department of Radiology, Huadu District People's Hospital of Guangzhou, Guangzhou, Guangdong, People's Republic of China

Hui-Li Zhan Department of Radiology, Beijing Jishuitan Hospital, Beijing, People's Republic of China

Bu-Tian Zhang Department of Radiology, People's Republic of China-Japan Union Hospital, Jilin University, Changchun, Jilin, People's Republic of China

Jing Zhang Department of Radiology, Beijing Jishuitan Hospital, Beijing, People's Republic of China

Yan Zhang Department of Radiology, Ordos Central Hospital, Ordos, Inner Mongolia, People's Republic of China

Yong-Hua Zhang Department of Radiology, Dalian Municipal Center Hospital, Dalian Medical University, Dalian, Liaoning, People's Republic of China

Feng Zhao Department of Radiology, Shaoxing People's Hospital, Shaoxing, Zhejiang, People's Republic of China

Xiao-Sen Zhou Department of Radiology, People's Hospital of Zunhua, Zunhua, Hebei, People's Republic of China

Part I

Hip

Aneurysmal Bone Cyst: Case 1

1.1   Medical History

An 18-year-old male with right thigh pain for 6 days after a fall.

1.2   Physical Examination

Point tenderness at the right proximal femur.

1.3   Imaging Findings

1.3.1   Radiograph

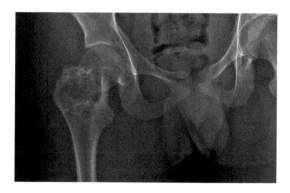

Fig. 1.1 Frontal view of the right hip

© Springer Nature Singapore Pte Ltd. and Peking Union Medical College Press 2020
X. Cheng et al., *Bone Tumor Imaging*, https://doi.org/10.1007/978-981-13-9927-5_1

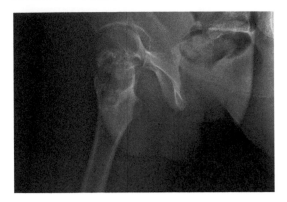

Fig. 1.2 Frog leg lateral view of the right hip

Radiographs of the right hip demonstrate an expansile, bubbly lucent lesion in the right femoral neck and extend to the intertrochanteric region, with internal septations. The medial rim of the lesion is sclerotic.

1.3.2   CT Imaging

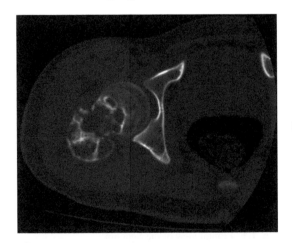

Fig. 1.3 Axial CT scan of the right hip in bone window

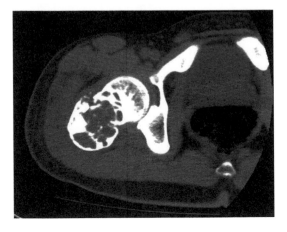

Fig. 1.4 Axial CT scan of the right hip in soft tissue window

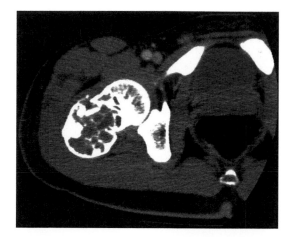

Fig. 1.5 Axial post-contrast CT scan of the right hip in soft tissue window

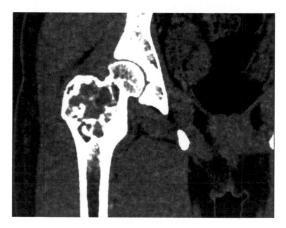

Fig. 1.6 Coronal post-contrast CT scan of the right hip in soft tissue window

CT images of the right hip demonstrate a lytic lesion with multiple large, irregular internal septations and peripheral sclerosis involving the right femoral neck and extending to the intertrochanteric region. There is marked enhancement surrounding the septations and along the borders.

1.3.3 MR Imaging

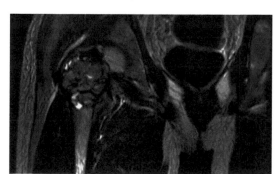

Fig. 1.7 Coronal T2-weighted MR image of the right hip

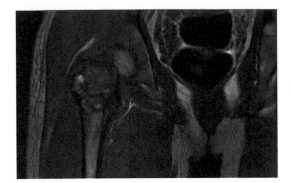

Fig. 1.8 Coronal T1-weighted MR image of the right hip

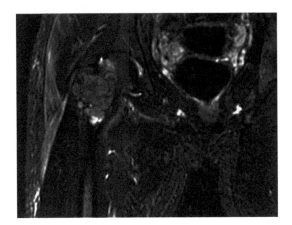

Fig. 1.9 Coronal fat-suppressed T2-weighted MR image of the right hip

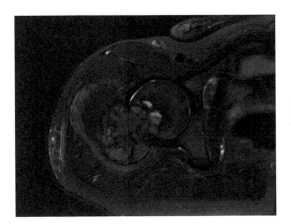

Fig. 1.10 Axial fat-suppressed T2-weighted MR image of the right hip

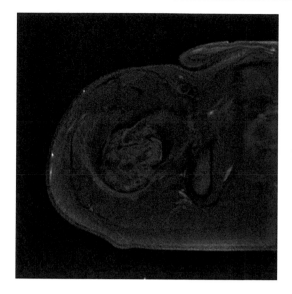

Fig. 1.11 Axial fat-suppressed, post-contrast T1-weighted MR image of the right hip

MR images of the right hip demonstrate multiple fluid-fluid levels within the lesion with septal enhancement.

1.4   Description and Discussion from Residents

The patient is an adolescent male. The radiographs of right hip demonstrate a lesion in the proximal right femur, which is mildly expansile with slightly indistinct border. The lesion has a bubbly appearance, due to the multiple internal bony septations. There is a transverse lucent line noted in the medial cortex of the femoral neck, indicating pathologic fracture. CT images confirmed the presence of many internal bony septations and the sclerotic rim. The enhancement of soft tissues surrounding the septations and at border are noted on the post-contrast CT images. MR images demonstrate the characteristic feature of multiple fluid-fluid levels within the lesion. The combination of the above findings is highly suggestive of aneurysmal bone cyst (ABC) with pathological fracture.

1.5   Analysis and Comments from Professor Cheng Xiao-Guang

The patient is an adolescent male with history of fall. A translucent fracture line at the proximal right femur is visible on the radiographs. Well-defined sclerotic rim and multiple internal septations are also seen on the radiographs, which are typical for benign bone lesions. CT images clearly demonstrate the sclerotic rim and multiple internal septations, but with no internal matrix mineralization. MR images demonstrate this lesion contains multiple fluid-fluid levels. Additionally, there are many small high-signal areas within the lesion on T1-weighted images, which implies hemorrhage. There is also septal enhancement noted on both CT and MRI post-contrast images. Based on the above findings, primary ABC or secondary ABC to a benign lesion is at the top of the differential diagnosis. Statistically, giant cell tumor (GCT) and chondroblastoma are the most common lesions in the greater trochanteric region. However, GCT is unlikely in this case, because GCT lacks the bony septations. Chondroblastoma generally causes significant bone marrow edema and surrounding tissue edema, whereas the perilesional edema in this case is insignificant. However, since edema may not be present in all cases of chondroblastoma, it does not necessarily exclude the diagnosis of chondroblastoma with ABC. Although the primary ABC could have identical radiographic appearances, its occurrence in the greater trochanter is relatively rare. Therefore, chondroblastoma with ABC would be the most likely diagnosis in this case.

1.6 Diagnosis

Aneurysmal bone cyst with pathological fracture.

Suggested Reading

Kransdorf MJ, Sweet DE. Aneurysmal bone cyst: concept, controversy, clinical presentation, and imaging. AJR Am J Roentgenol. 1995;164(3):573–80.

Van Dyck P, Vanhoenacker FM, Vogel J, et al. Prevalence, extension and characteristics of fluid-fluid levels in bone and soft tissue tumors. Eur Radiol. 2006;16(12):2644–51.

Aneurysmal Bone Cyst: Case 2

2

2.1   Medical History

A 29-year-old male with left hip pain, discomfort, and decreased range of motion for 9 months and worsening limping for 2 months.

2.2   Physical Examination

No focal swelling around the left hip with normal skin temperature. No palpable mass.

2.3   Imaging Findings

2.3.1   Radiograph

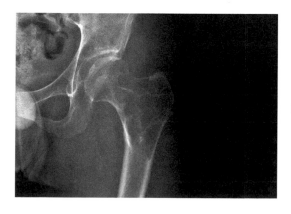

Fig. 2.1 Frontal view of the left hip

© Springer Nature Singapore Pte Ltd. and Peking Union Medical College Press 2020
X. Cheng et al., *Bone Tumor Imaging*, https://doi.org/10.1007/978-981-13-9927-5_2

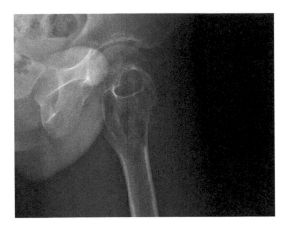

Fig. 2.2 Frog leg lateral view of the left hip

Radiographs of the left hip demonstrate an
expansile, lytic lesion in the left proximal femur
with well-defined margin and no sclerosis.

2.3.2 CT Imaging

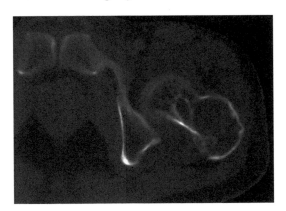

Fig. 2.3 Axial CT scan of the left hip in bone window

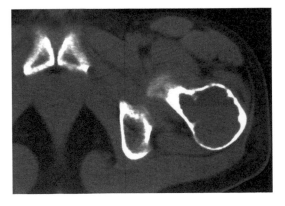

Fig. 2.4 Axial CT scan of the left hip in soft tissue
window

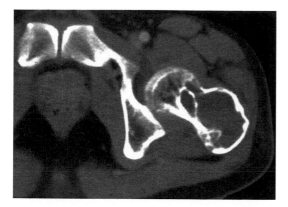

Fig. 2.5 Axial post-contrast CT scan of the left hip in soft tissue window

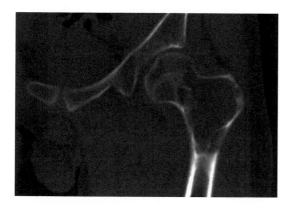

Fig. 2.6 Coronal CT scan of the left hip in bone window

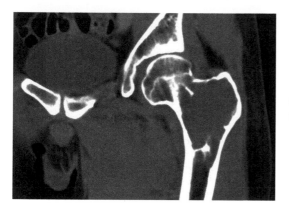

Fig. 2.7 Coronal post-contrast CT scan of the left hip in soft tissue window

CT images of the left hip demonstrate well-defined margin of the lytic lesion with internal heterogeneous density. There are internal bone septation, fluid-fluid level with cortical break of the anterior cortex.

2.3.3 MR Imaging

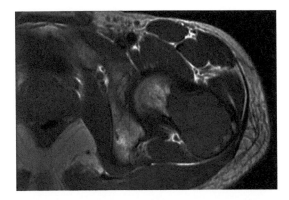

Fig. 2.8 Axial T1-weighted MR image of the left hip

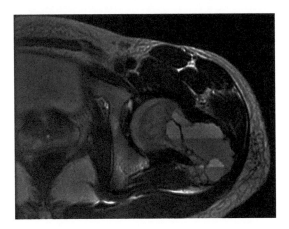

Fig. 2.9 Axial T2-weighted MR image of the left hip

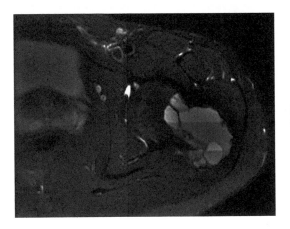

Fig. 2.10 Axial fat-suppressed T2-weighted MR image of the left hip

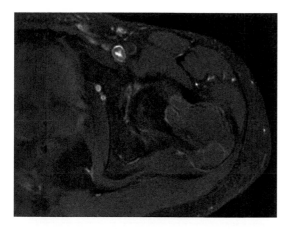

Fig. 2.11   Axial fat-suppressed post-contrast T1-weighted MR image of the left hip

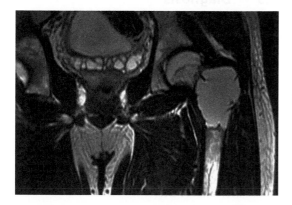

Fig. 2.12   Coronal T2-weighted MR image of the left hip

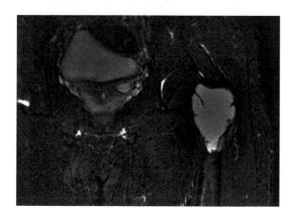

Fig. 2.13   Coronal fat-suppressed T2-weighted MR image of the left hip

MR images of the left hip demonstrate multiple fluid-fluid levels within the lytic lesion. And there is mild peripheral enhancement.

2.4 Description and Discussion from Residents

The patient is a young adult male. The radiographs of the left hip demonstrate a lytic lesion in the proximal left femur. The lesion has well-defined margin and internal septations with thinning of the cortex and mildly expansile. On the CT scan, there is predominantly internal fluid density without calcification or soft tissue mass. Also, there is a cortical break with some soft tissue protuberance and no clear enhancement. Multiple fluid-fluid levels, some are more broad based on MR images. Mild surrounding edema is also noted. The diagnosis is likely to be aneurysmal bone cyst (ABC).

2.5 Analysis and Comments from Professor Cheng Xiao-Guang

The patient is a young adult male. There is a lytic lesion in the proximal femur involving the greater trochanteric and intertrochanteric region without sclerosis. There is no calcification noted on soft tissue window of CT scan images. However, aggressive lesion cannot be excluded due to focal cortical break, such as telangiectatic osteosarcoma. Though, no enhancement is seen on CT images. There is a clear low T1 signal on T1-weighted images and multiple fluid-fluid levels on T2-weighted images. When more percentage of the lesion is covered by fluid-fluid levels, it is more likely to be benign. Given the above combination of findings, benign lesion such as aneurysmal bone cyst is the favored diagnosis.

2.6 Diagnosis

Aneurysmal bone cyst.

Suggested Reading

Kransdorf MJ, Sweet DE. Aneurysmal bone cyst: concept, controversy, clinical presentation, and imaging. AJR Am J Roentgenol. 1995;164(3):573–80.

Van Dyck P, Vanhoenacker FM, Vogel J, et al. Prevalence, extension and characteristics of fluid-fluid levels in bone and soft tissue tumors. Eur Radiol. 2006;16(12):2644–51.

Osteoid Osteoma: Case 3

3.1 Medical History

A 15-year-old boy with left hip pain and decreased range of motion for 4 months, exacerbates at night.

3.2 Physical Examination

Swelling around the left hip with mild tenderness and restricted range of motion.

3.3 Imaging Findings

3.3.1 Radiograph

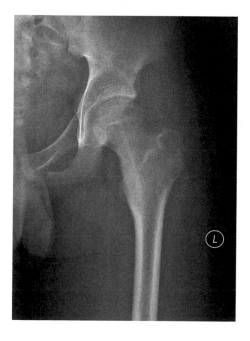

Fig. 3.1 Frontal view of the left hip

© Springer Nature Singapore Pte Ltd. and Peking Union Medical College Press 2020
X. Cheng et al., *Bone Tumor Imaging*, https://doi.org/10.1007/978-981-13-9927-5_3

Radiograph of the left hip shows subtle cortical thickening around the left proximal femur in the medial aspect.

3.3.2   CT Imaging

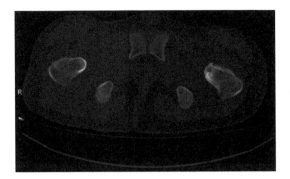

Fig. 3.2 Axial CT scan of the left hip in bone window

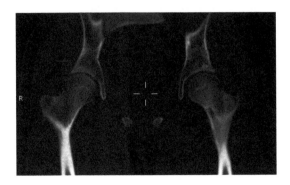

Fig. 3.3 Coronal CT scan of the left hip in bone window

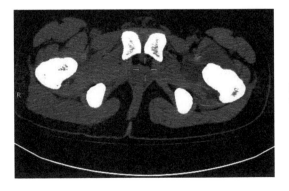

Fig. 3.4 Axial CT scan of the left hip in soft tissue window

CT images of the left hip demonstrate cortical thickening around the medial cortex of the left femoral neck and lesser trochanter. There is a small internal lucent nidus.

3.4 Description and Discussion from Residents

There is a subtle cortical thickening around the medial cortex of the left proximal femur with the suggestion of internal low density on radiograph. The cortical thickening is better delineated on CT scan with internal semicircle low density and calcification. There is also periosteal reaction with edema of the surrounding soft tissue. The combination of the findings is consistent with osteoid osteoma.

3.5 Analysis and Comments from Professor Cheng Xiao-Guang

The imaging features of cortical thickening along the medial cortex of the left femoral neck with internal nidus and surrounding reactive sclerosis, soft tissue edema, and swelling around the joint are all characteristic findings for osteoid osteoma.

3.6 Diagnosis

Osteoid osteoma.

Suggested Reading

Chai JW, Hong SH, Choi JY, et al. Radiologic diagnosis of osteoid osteoma: from simple to challenging findings. Radiographics. 2010;30(3):737–49.

Touraine S, Emerich L, Bisseret D, et al. Is pain duration associated with morphologic changes of osteoid osteomas at CT? Radiology. 2014;271(3):795–804.

Osteoid Osteoma: Case 4

4

4.1　Medical History

A 7-year-old girl presented with right hip pain for 7 months and limping for 4 months.

4.2　Physical Examination

Limping of the right lower extremity. There is smaller circumference of the right thigh compared to the left. No tenderness around the right hip.

4.3　Imaging Findings

4.3.1　Radiograph

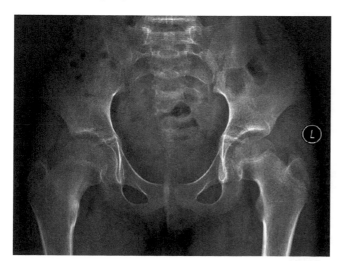

Fig. 4.1 Frontal view of the right hip

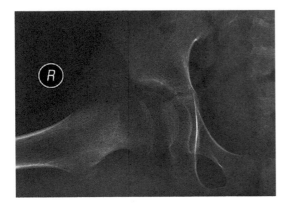

Fig. 4.2 Frog lateral view of the right hip

Radiographs of the right hip demonstrate cortical thickening of the medial cortex of the right femoral neck with internal low density.

4.3.2   CT Imaging

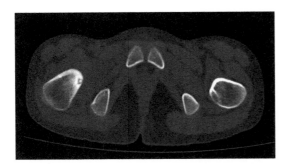

Fig. 4.3 Axial CT scan of the right hip in bone window

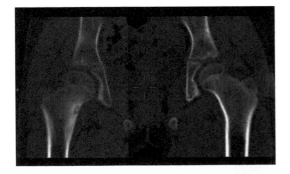

Fig. 4.4 Coronal CT scan of the right hip in bone window

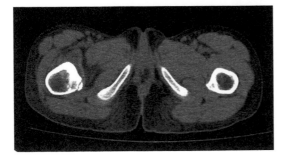

Fig. 4.5 Axial CT scan of the right hip in soft tissue window

CT images of the right hip demonstrate cortical thickening around the medial cortex of the right femoral neck with internal small round low-density nidus with calcification. There is swelling in the surrounding soft tissue.

4.4 Description and Discussion from Residents

There is cortical thickening around the medial cortex of the right femoral neck on radiographs. CT scan shows internal semicircular low density with foci of calcification and surrounding reactive sclerosis and soft tissue edema. The combination of the findings is consistent with osteoid osteoma.

4.5 Analysis and Comments from Professor Cheng Xiao-Guang

There is semicircular low-density nidus with foci of calcification and surrounding reactive sclerosis around the right femoral neck. The femoral neck lacks external periosteum, so there is no periosteal reaction. With the presence of surrounding soft tissue edema and joint effusion, osteoid osteoma is the favored diagnosis with typical imaging findings.

4.6 Diagnosis

Osteoid osteoma.

Suggested Reading

Chai JW, Hong SH, Choi JY, et al. Radiologic diagnosis of osteoid osteoma: from simple to challenging findings. Radiographics. 2010;30(3):737–49.

Kransdorf MJ, Stull MA, Gilkey FW, et al. Osteoid osteoma. Radiographics. 1991;11(4):671–96.

Osteochondroma: Case 5

5.1 Medical History

A 29-year-old male presented with left hip pain and discomfort for more than a year and worse for the last 3 months.

5.2 Physical Examination

Palpable hard mass around the left hip joint.

5.3 Imaging Findings

5.3.1 Radiograph

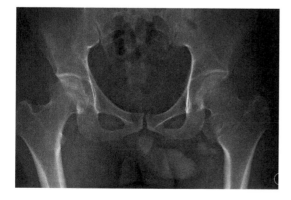

Fig. 5.1 Frontal view of the left hip

© Springer Nature Singapore Pte Ltd. and Peking Union Medical College Press 2020
X. Cheng et al., *Bone Tumor Imaging*, https://doi.org/10.1007/978-981-13-9927-5_5

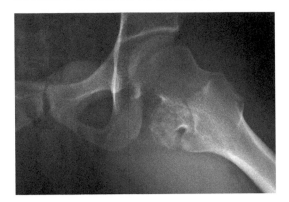

Fig. 5.2 Frog lateral view of the left hip

Radiographs of the left hip demonstrate an exostosis along the medial cortex of the left femoral neck in a cauliflower-like morphology with broad base and medullary continuity. There is external irregularity of the lesion with surrounding several small ossific densities.

5.3.2 CT Imaging

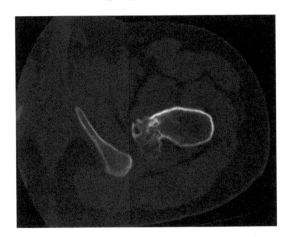

Fig. 5.3 Axial CT scan of the left hip in bone window

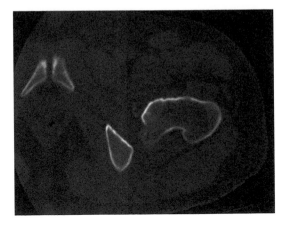

Fig. 5.4 Axial CT scan of the left hip in bone window

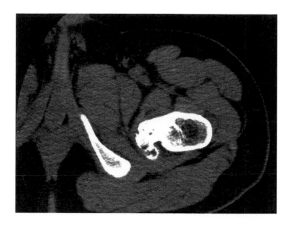

Fig. 5.5 Axial CT scan of the left hip in soft tissue window

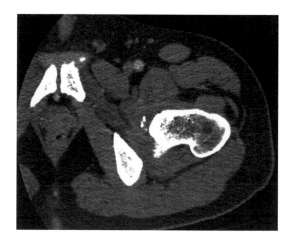

Fig. 5.6 Axial CT scan of the post-contrast left hip in soft tissue window

CT images of the left hip clearly demonstrate similar findings as seen on the radiograph. There are soft tissue densities at the peripheral of the lesion.

5.4 Description and Discussion from Residents

The patient is a young male. There is an exostosis along the left femoral neck and lesser trochanter with cortical and medullary continuity, typical of osteochondroma.

5.5 Analysis and Comments from Professor Cheng Xiao-Guang

The patient is a young male. With the presence of an exostosis along the left femoral neck and lesser trochanter and cortical and medullary continuity, osteochondroma is at the top of the differential diagnosis. However, several ossific densities noted around the lesion raise the concern for calcification around the cartilaginous cap versus fracture around the cartilage after injury. Given there is soft tissue of low density noted around the lesion on CT scan, MRI is recommended to better evaluate the surrounding soft tissue and exclude the possibility of malignant transformation.

5.6   Diagnosis

Osteochondroma.

Suggested Reading

Ahmed AR, Tan TS, Unni KK et al. Secondary chondrosarcoma in osteochondroma: report of 107 patients. Clin Orthop Relat Res. 2003;(411):193–206.

Bernard SA, Murphey MD, Flemming DJ, et al. Improved differentiation of benign osteochondromas from secondary chondrosarcomas with standardized measurement of cartilage cap at CT and MR imaging. Radiology. 2010;255(3):857–65.

Chondroblastoma: Recurrence Case 6

6

6.1 Medical History

An 8-year-old boy presented with right hip pain after jumping down from bed about 1 year and 9 months ago. He underwent curettage of the femoral head with graft placement. About 1 month ago, the patient started to experience paroxysmal pain around the right hip.

6.2 Physical Examination

Limping. Restricted squatting. Scar around the right inguinal region and along the right iliac crest.

6.3 Imaging Findings

6.3.1 Radiograph

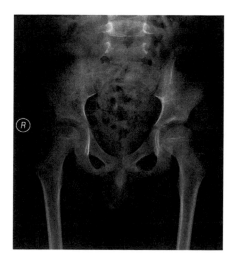

Fig. 6.1 Frontal view of the right hip

© Springer Nature Singapore Pte Ltd. and Peking Union Medical College Press 2020
X. Cheng et al., *Bone Tumor Imaging*, https://doi.org/10.1007/978-981-13-9927-5_6

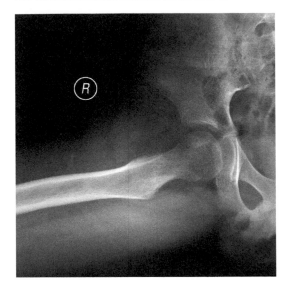

Fig. 6.2 Frog lateral view of the right hip

Radiographs of the right hip demonstrate asymmetric low-density lesion along the epiphysis of the right femoral head with clear margin and slight expansile appearance.

6.3.2   CT Imaging

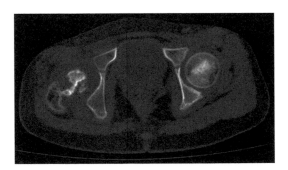

Fig. 6.3 Axial CT scan of the right hip in bone window

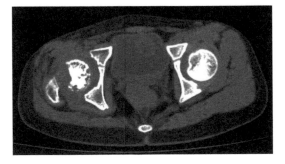

Fig. 6.4 Axial CT scan of the right hip in soft tissue window

CT images of the right hip demonstrate irregular bony destruction along the right femoral head with internal numerous, sandy like calcifications. There is also right hip joint effusion.

6.3.3 MR Imaging

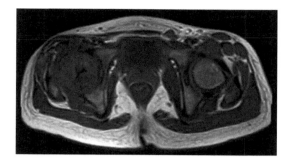

Fig. 6.5 Axial T1-weighted MR image of the right hip

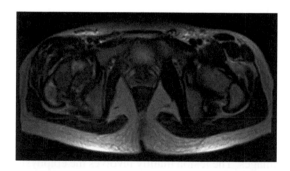

Fig. 6.6 Axial T2-weighted MR image of the right hip

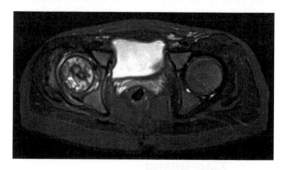

Fig. 6.7 Axial fat-suppressed T2-weighted MR image of the right hip

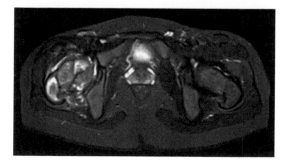

Fig. 6.8 Axial fat-suppressed T2-weighted MR image of the right hip

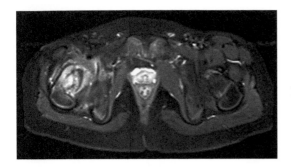

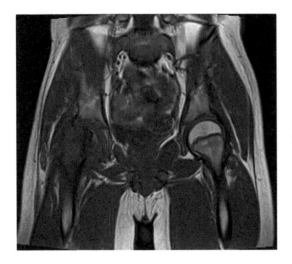

Fig. 6.9 Axial fat-suppressed post-contrast T1-weighted MR image of the right hip

Fig. 6.10 Coronal T1-weighted MR image of the right hip

MR images of the right hip demonstrate heterogeneous signal of the lesion with surrounding soft tissue edema and associated enhancement.

6.4 Description and Discussion from Residents

There is bony destruction around the right femoral head epiphysis with clear margin on the radiographs. The joint space was relatively preserved with surrounding soft tissue swelling. The CT scan is about 1 year after the initial radiographs and demonstrates that the lesion has increased in size and now involves the femoral neck with ill-defined margin and internal high densities. There is continued preserved joint space. There is clear soft tissue edema on MR

images. The lesion mainly involves the epiphysis with history of surgery, and chondroblastoma recurrence is the favored diagnosis. Differential diagnosis: (1) Infectious etiology, usually affects the weight-bearing area with loss of joint space, not seen on the current study; (2) eosinophilic granuloma.

6.5 Analysis and Comments from Professor Cheng Xiao-Guang

There is well-defined destruction around the right femoral head epiphysis, which is typical for chondroblastoma on radiograph. There is a long time gap between the initial radiograph and the CT scan. There is no joint space loss. With the history of surgery and surrounding soft tissue edema on MR and solid signals inside of the lesion, infectious etiology can be excluded, and recurrence of chondroblastoma is favored.

6.6 Diagnosis

Chondroblastoma recurrence after surgery.

Suggested Reading

Ebeid WA, Hasan BZ, Badr IT, et al. Functional and oncological outcome after treatment of chondroblastoma with intralesional curettage. J Pediatr Orthop. 2019;39(4):e312–7.

Kaim AH, Hügli R, Bonél HM, et al. Chondroblastoma and clear cell chondrosarcoma radiological and MRI characteristics with histopathological correlation. Skelet Radiol. 2002;31(2):88–95.

7.1 Medical History

A 59-year-old male presented with right thigh pain for 3 months and worsened in the last 1 month.

7.2 Physical Examination

Swelling around the right hip joint with decreased range of motion and tenderness.

7.3 Imaging Findings

7.3.1 Radiograph

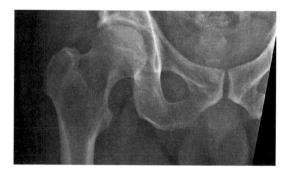

Fig. 7.1 Frontal view of the right hip

Radiograph of the right hip demonstrates a lucent lesion at the intertrochanteric region with ill-defined border. There is also swelling around the right hip joint.

7.3.2 CT Imaging

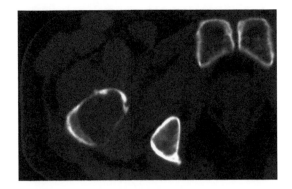

Fig. 7.2 Axial CT scan of the right hip in bone window

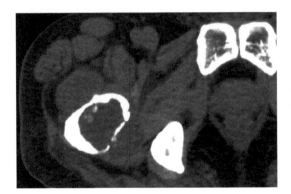

Fig. 7.3 Axial CT scan of the right hip in soft tissue window

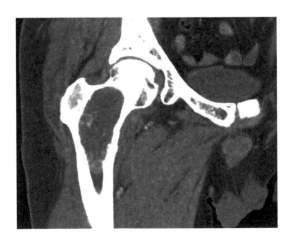

Fig. 7.4 Coronal post-contrast CT scan of the right hip in soft tissue window

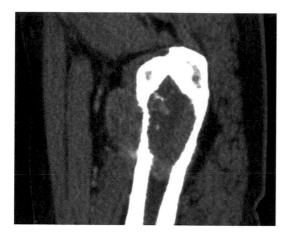

Fig. 7.5 Sagittal post-contrast CT scan of the right hip in soft tissue window

CT images of the right hip demonstrate bony destruction and associated soft tissue mass. There are internal scattered calcifications. On the post-contrast images, there are scattered nodular enhancements.

7.3.3 MR Imaging

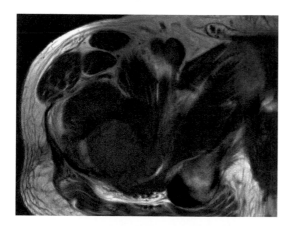

Fig. 7.6 Axial T1-weighted MR image of the right hip

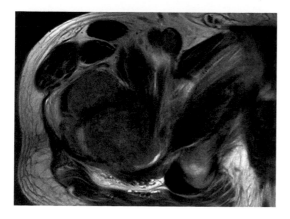

Fig. 7.7 Axial T2-weighted MR image of the right hip

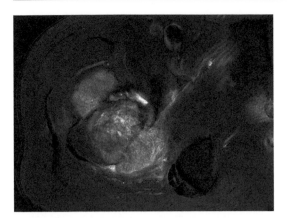

Fig. 7.8 Axial fat-suppressed T2-weighted MR image of the right hip

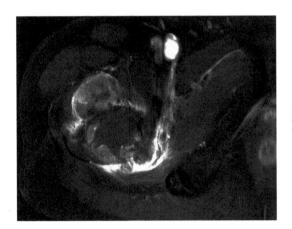

Fig. 7.9 Axial fat-suppressed post-contrast T1-weighted MR image of the right hip

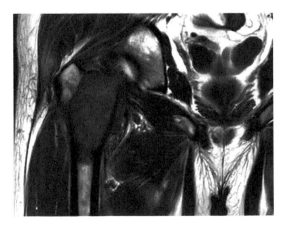

Fig. 7.10 Coronal T1-weighted MR image of the right hip

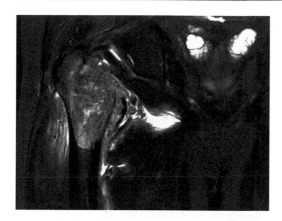

Fig. 7.11 Coronal fat-suppressed T2-weighted MR image of the right hip

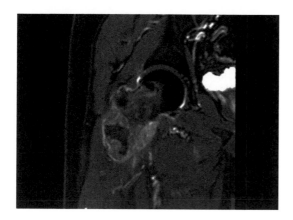

Fig. 7.12 Coronal fat-suppressed post-contrast T1-weighted MR image of the right hip

MR images of the right hip demonstrate heterogeneous signal of the lesion with a prominent soft tissue mass of extensive blood supply and heterogeneous enhancement.

7.4 Description and Discussion from Residents

There are lytic bony destructive changes around the proximal right femur with ill-defined margin on radiograph. CT scan again demonstrates the lytic bony destructive changes around the right proximal femur with destruction of the bony cortex. There are septation and calcification within the lesion and mildly aggressive features. There is associated enhancement. The above findings are suggestive of underlying chondroid matrix and possible chondrosarcoma; however, other malignant lesion such as malignant fibrous histiocytomas and metastatic lesion cannot be excluded.

7.5 Analysis and Comments from Professor Cheng Xiao-Guang

Radiograph demonstrates ill-defined lytic bony destructive changes around the right intertrochanteric region, suspicious for pathologic fracture. On CT images, there is an ill-defined lesion with cortical break, and the soft tissue mass extends beyond the cortex with internal nodular high densities, suspicious for calcification. After contrast, no definitive enhancement is noted in the region of bony destructive changes, but there is heterogeneous enhancement in the soft tissue mass. The MR images demonstrate the lesion in more detail with clear soft tissue mass and enhancement. With the above constellation of findings and patient's age, this is a malignant lesion. Differential diagnosis includes malignant fibrous histiocytomas, metastatic lesion, and chondrosarcoma. However, typically there is high T2 signal on T2-weighted images in cases of chondrosarcoma with subtle enhancement, not consistent with the current case.

7.6   Diagnosis

Alveolar soft part sarcoma.

Suggested Reading

Cao Y, Zhang H, Qu Y, et al. Primary alveolar soft part sarcoma of the right femur and primary lymphoma of the left femur: a case report and literature review. Oncol Lett. 2016;11(1):89–94.

Crombé A, Brisse HJ, Ledoux P, et al. Alveolar soft-part sarcoma: can MRI help discriminating from other soft-tissue tumors? A study of the French sarcoma group. Eur Radiol. 2019;29(6):3170–82. https://doi.org/10.1007/s00330-018-5903-3.

McCarville MB, Muzzafar S, Kao SC, et al. Imaging features of alveolar soft-part sarcoma: a report from children's oncology group study ARST0332. AJR Am J Roentgenol. 2014;203(6):1345–52.

Chondromyxoid Fibroma: Case 8

8.1 Medical History

A 21-year-old male presented with right hip discomfort for about half a year.

8.2 Physical Examination

Mild atrophy of the right lower extremity compared to the left. Mild swelling around the proximal right thigh with palpable mass. The palpable mass is hard with point tenderness but no clear margin.

8.3 Imaging Findings

8.3.1 Radiograph

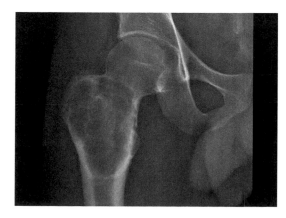

Fig. 8.1 Frontal view of the right hip

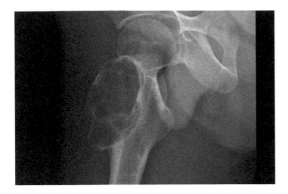

Fig. 8.2 Lateral view of the right hip

Radiographs of the right hip demonstrate a low density with clear margin. There are internal heterogeneous densities and thick septations.

8.3.2   CT Imaging

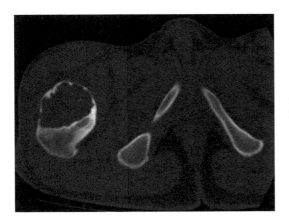

Fig. 8.3 Axial CT scan of the right proximal femur in bone window

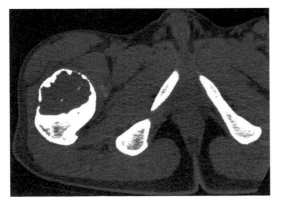

Fig. 8.4 Axial CT scan of the right proximal femur in soft tissue window

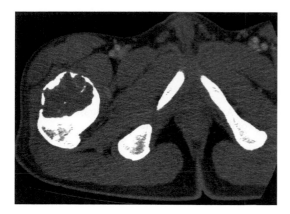

Fig. 8.5 Axial post-contrast CT scan of the right proximal femur in soft tissue window

CT images of the proximal right femur demonstrate bony destruction of the right femoral neck and greater trochanter. There are internal high densities with focal cortical break. The cortical margin demonstrates a "scalloped" appearance with heterogeneous mild enhancement.

8.3.3 MR Imaging

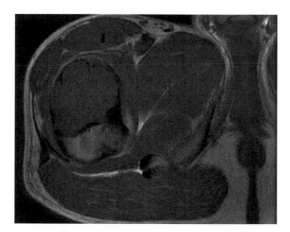

Fig. 8.6 Axial T1-weighted MR image of the right proximal femur

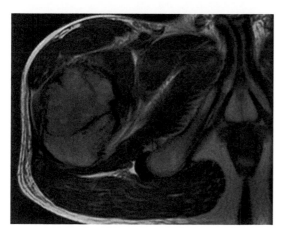

Fig. 8.7 Axial T2-weighted MR image of the right proximal femur

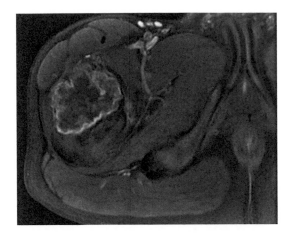

Fig. 8.8 Axial fat-suppressed post-contrast T1-weighted image of the right proximal femur

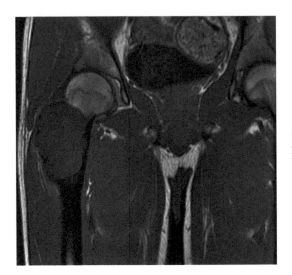

Fig. 8.9 Coronal T1-weighted MR image of the right proximal femur

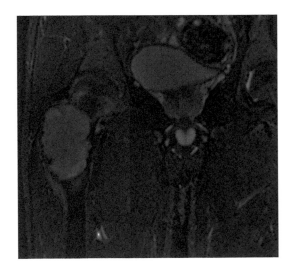

Fig. 8.10 Coronal fat-suppressed T2-weighted MR image of the right proximal femur

MR images of the right proximal femur demonstrate there is predominant high T2 signal within the bony destructive lesion. There are bony septations around the margin and peripheral enhancement.

8.4 Description and Discussion from Residents

There are expansile bony destructive changes around the right proximal femur with peripheral sclerosis and internal septations. There is no associated soft tissue mass or periosteal reaction. These features are most suggestive of a benign bone tumor, such as aneurysmal bone cyst (ABC) or giant cell tumor. CT images demonstrate clear margin of the lesion with peripheral sclerosis, internal scattered high densities, and without fluid-fluid level, most suggestive of a benign lesion. On MR images, there is isointense T1 signal and heterogeneous high T2 signal and heterogeneous enhancement, most suggestive of benign chondroid lesion or low-grade malignant lesion.

8.5 Analysis and Comments from Professor Cheng Xiao-Guang

Radiographs demonstrate well-defined bony destructive changes along the right proximal femur with peripheral sclerosis, most suggestive of benign lesion, such as chondroblastoma or giant cell tumor. Peripheral scalloped appearances with internal isolated point calcification are noted on CT images. There is isointense T1 and high T2 signals with peripheral enhancement on MR images. High T2 signal suggests internal myxoid component. CT findings suggest chondroid matrix. The lesion is adjacent to the greater trochanter. Based on all the above features, it is likely to be chondromyxoid fibroma. Differential diagnosis includes chondroblastoma. However, if this is a chondroblastoma and with the large size, usually there are cystic changes which are not present on the current case.

8.6 Diagnosis

Chondromyxoid fibroma.

Suggested Reading

Kim HS, Jee WH, Ryu KN, et al. MRI of chondromyxoid fibroma. Acta Radiol. 2011;52(8):875–80.

Wu CT, Inwards CY, O'Laughlin S, et al. Chondromyxoid fibroma of bone: a clinicopathologic review of 278 cases. Hum Pathol. 1998;29(5):438–46.

9.1 Medical History

A 6-year-old girl presented with mass around the left gluteal region for 2 years with prior history of surgery.

9.2 Physical Examination

Palpable hard mass at the left gluteal region without point tenderness.

9.3 Imaging Findings

9.3.1 MR Imaging

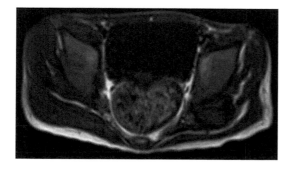

Fig. 9.1 Axial T1-weighted MR image of the left gluteal region

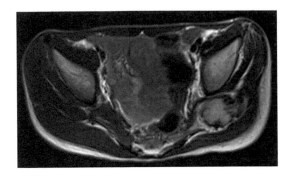

Fig. 9.2 Axial T2-weighted MR image of the left gluteal region

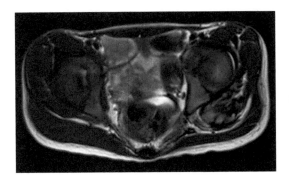

Fig. 9.3 Axial T2-weighted MR image of the left gluteal region

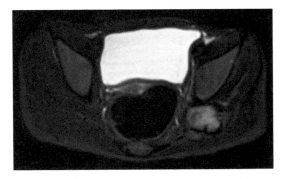

Fig. 9.4 Axial fat-suppressed T2-weighted MR image of the left gluteal region

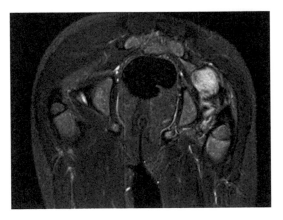

Fig. 9.5 Coronal fat-suppressed T2-weighted MR image of the left gluteal region

MR images demonstrate abnormal signal involving the left gluteus medius and gluteus minimus muscles with isointense T1 and mildly high T2 signals. The lesion shows irregular border without clear margin from surrounding musculatures. There are low signal septations on T2-weighted images with heterogeneous enhancement.

9.4 Description and Discussion from Residents

There is a soft tissue mass in the left gluteal region with isointense T1 and slightly high T2 signals with clear border and no adjacent soft tissue invasion. Given the long duration of the symptoms and above imaging features, this is likely to be a benign lesion. There is linear low signal in the lesion, most suggestive of desmoid-type fibromatosis. Differential diagnoses include hemangioma which usually shows high signal, or nerve sheath tumor which usually follows the neurovascular bundle.

9.5 Analysis and Comments from Professor Cheng Xiao-Guang

Linear low signal within the soft tissue mass on MR images are most suggestive of desmoid-type fibromatosis. Desmoid fibromatosis tends to involve the gluteal region, highly invasive with high recurrence rate. Given there is gluteal muscle atrophy, gluteal muscle contracture must be excluded. This is best evaluated with GRE sequence and usually caused by local injection. Soft tissue mass seen of the current case excluded the possibility of gluteal muscle contracture.

9.6 Diagnosis

Desmoid-type fibromatosis.

Suggested Reading

Gondim Teixeira PA, Chanson A, Verhaeghe JL, et al. Correlation between tumor growth and hormonal therapy with MR signal characteristics of desmoid-type fibromatosis: a preliminary study. Diagn Interv Imaging. 2019;100(1):47–55.

Otero S, Moskovic EC, Strauss DC. Desmoid-type fibromatosis. Clin Radiol. 2015;70(9):1038–45.

Robbin MR, Murphey MD, Temple HT, et al. Imaging of musculoskeletal fibromatosis. Radiographics. 2001;21(3):585–600.

10.1 Medical History

A 3-year-old girl presented with pain around the right gluteal region for 1 year and limping for 3 months. She was diagnosed with "gluteal muscle contracture" and treated with surgery.

10.2 Physical Examination

Limping. Scar tissue around the posterior lateral right gluteal region from prior surgery. Palpable hard mass with point tenderness. Decreased range of motion of the right hip joint.

10.3 Imaging Findings

10.3.1 MR Imaging

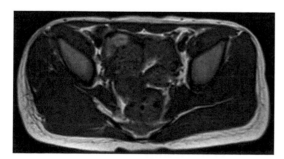

Fig. 10.1 Axial T1-weighted MR image of the right gluteal region

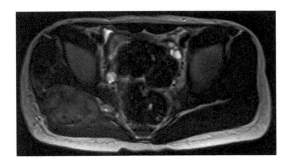

Fig. 10.2 Axial T2-weighted MR image of the right gluteal region

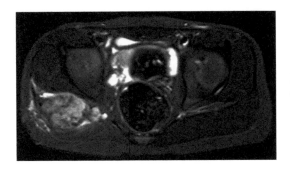

Fig. 10.3 Axial fat-suppressed T2-weighted MR image of the right gluteal region

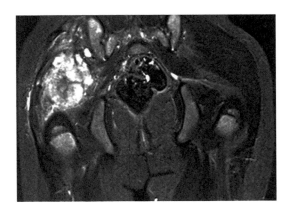

Fig. 10.4 Coronal fat-suppressed T2-weighted MR image of the right gluteal region

MR images demonstrate focal isointense T1 and high T2 signals soft tissue mass within the left gluteus maximus and gluteus medius muscles. There are internal linear low T1 and low T2 signals.

10.4   Description and Discussion from Residents

There is a soft tissue mass in the right gluteal region. There are internal septations with low T2 signal, most suggestive of desmoid-type fibromatosis. The imaging features are very similar to

Case 9. The only difference is the presence of extensive surrounding soft tissue edema, likely due to prior surgery.

10.5   Analysis and Comments from Professor Cheng Xiao-Guang

Like Case 9, there is a high signal in the soft tissue mass on fat-suppressed sequence with internal linear low signals, most suggestive of desmoid-type fibromatosis. The lesion was not entirely excised even with prior surgery.

10.6 Diagnosis

Desmoid-type fibromatosis.

Suggested Reading

Gondim Teixeira PA, Chanson A, Verhaeghe JL, et al. Correlation between tumor growth and hormonal therapy with MR signal characteristics of desmoid-type fibromatosis: a preliminary study. Diagn Interv Imaging. 2019;100(1):47–55.

Otero S, Moskovic EC, Strauss DC. Desmoid-type fibromatosis. Clin Radiol. 2015;70(9):1038–45.

Robbin MR, Murphey MD, Temple HT, et al. Imaging of musculoskeletal fibromatosis. Radiographics. 2001;21(3):585–600.

Giant Cell Tumor of Bone: Case 11

11

11.1 Medical History

A 29-year-old female presented with right hip pain and restricted activities for 3 year and worsened in the last 2 months. She had a history of prior surgery from her local hospital.

11.2 Physical Examination

Focal mass without clear border, hard, with point tenderness.

11.3 Imaging Findings

11.3.1 Radiograph

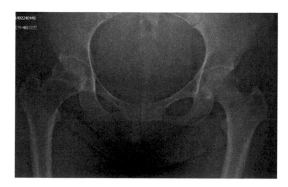

Fig. 11.1 Frontal view of the right hip

© Springer Nature Singapore Pte Ltd. and Peking Union Medical College Press 2020
X. Cheng et al., *Bone Tumor Imaging*, https://doi.org/10.1007/978-981-13-9927-5_11

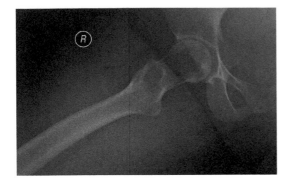

Fig. 11.2 Frog lateral view of the right hip

Radiographs of the right hip demonstrate lytic bony destructive changes of right femoral head and neck with focal cortical expansion and thinning. There is a clear margin of the lesion without sclerosis. Sequelae from prior surgery are noted.

11.3.2 CT Imaging

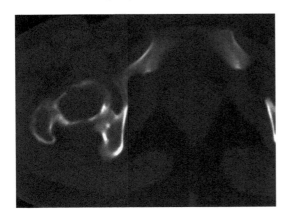

Fig. 11.3 Axial CT scan of the right hip in bone window

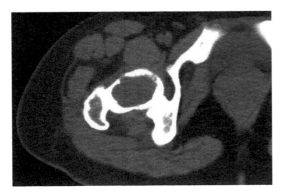

Fig. 11.4 Axial CT scan of the right hip in soft tissue window

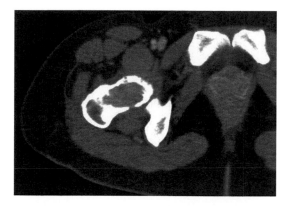

Fig. 11.5 Axial post-contrast CT scan of the right hip in soft tissue window

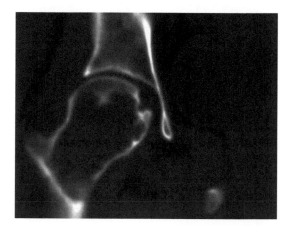

Fig. 11.6 Coronal CT scan of the right hip in bone window

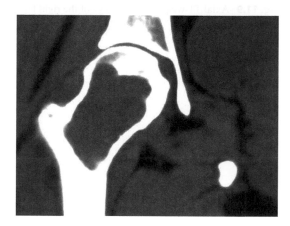

Fig. 11.7 Coronal CT scan of the right hip in soft tissue window

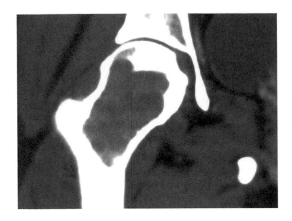

Fig. 11.8 Coronal post-contrast CT scan of the right hip in soft tissue window

CT images of the right hip demonstrate a well-defined lesion with cystic appearance and internal relatively homogeneous densities with clear enhancement. There is no associated soft tissue mass.

11.3.3 MR Imaging

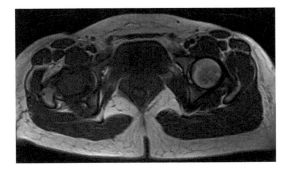

Fig. 11.9 Axial T1-weighted MR image of the right hip

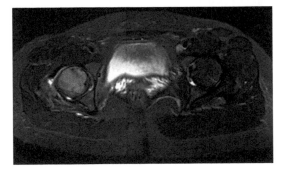

Fig. 11.10 Axial fat-suppressed T2-weighted MR image of the right hip

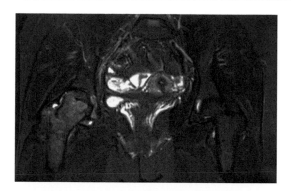

Fig. 11.11 Coronal fat-suppressed T2-weighted MR image of the right hip

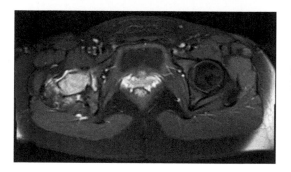

Fig. 11.12 Axial fat-suppressed post-contrast T1-weighted MR image of the right hip

MR images of the right hip demonstrate low T1 signal and mildly high T2 signal on fat-suppressed sequences of the lesion with avid enhancement.

11.4 Description and Discussion from Residents

There are lytic bony destructive changes of the right femoral neck without peripheral sclerosis but well-defined margin on radiographs. Prior screw tracks are noted of the right proximal femur, consistent with prior history of surgery. CT images demonstrate clear border of the lesion with some focal peripheral sclerosis and cortical discontinuities of the posterior cortex, without soft tissue mass or periosteal reaction. There are some internal scattered point and patchy high densities, likely representing calcification or bone fragments. There is avid enhancement. There is low T1 signal and high T2 signal of the

lesion on MR images with solid enhancement. All the above findings point to the diagnosis of giant cell tumor. However, with the internal high densities of likely calcification, differential diagnoses include cartilage tumors, such as chondroblastoma and clear cell chondrosarcoma.

11.5 Analysis and Comments from Professor Cheng Xiao-Guang

Given the short interval of recurrent symptoms, malignant transformation needs to be first excluded. However, there is a clear border on imaging; even with signs of low-grade invasiveness, this lesion likely favors to be benign. There is avid enhancement, most suggestive of recurrent giant cell tumor. Without typical focal chondroid matrix on MR images, chondroid lesion would not be included in the differential diagnosis.

11.6   Diagnosis

Giant cell tumor of bone.

Suggested Reading

Chakarun CJ, Forrester DM, Gottsegen CJ, et al. Giant cell tumor of bone: review, mimics, and new developments in treatment. Radiographics. 2013;33(1):197–211.

Klenke FM, Wenger DE, Inwards CY, et al. Giant cell tumor of bone: risk factors for recurrence. Clin Orthop Relat Res. 2011;469(2):591–9.

Murphey MD, Nomikos GC, Flemming DJ, et al. From the archives of AFIP. Imaging of giant cell tumor and giant cell reparative granuloma of bone: radiologic-pathologic correlation. Radiographics. 2001;21(5):1283–309.

12.1 Medical History

A 47-year-old male with right hip pain for one and half years and restricted range of motion for a year.

12.2 Physical Examination

Decreased range of motion of the right hip with normal strength.

12.3 Imaging Findings

12.3.1 MR Imaging

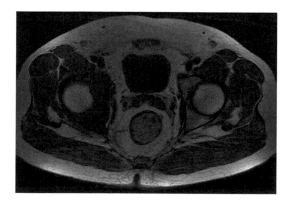

Fig. 12.1 Axial T1-weighted MR image of the right hip

© Springer Nature Singapore Pte Ltd. and Peking Union Medical College Press 2020
X. Cheng et al., *Bone Tumor Imaging*, https://doi.org/10.1007/978-981-13-9927-5_12

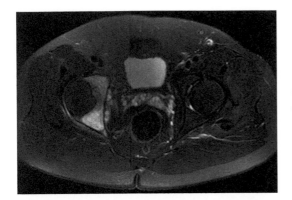

Fig. 12.2 Axial fat-suppressed T2-weighted MR image of the right hip

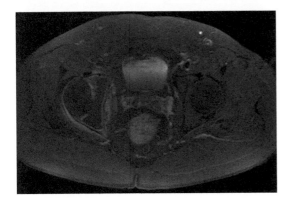

Fig. 12.3 Axial fat-suppressed post-contrast T1-weighted MR image of the right hip

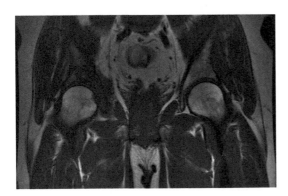

Fig. 12.4 Coronal T1-weighted MR image of the right hip

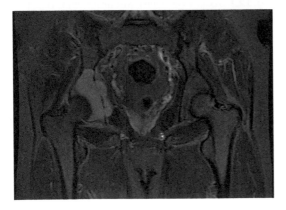

Fig. 12.5 Coronal fat-suppressed T2-weighted MR image of the right hip

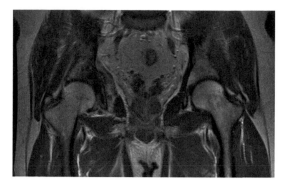

Fig. 12.6 Coronal post-contrast T1-weighted MR image of the right hip

MR images of the right hip demonstrate abnormal signal involving the right acetabulum with low T1 and high T2 signals and peripheral enhancement. There is a soft tissue mass along the medial wall of the right acetabulum with lobular enhancement.

12.4 Description and Discussion from Residents

MR images demonstrate abnormal signals involving the right acetabulum with low T1 and high T2 signals. There are focal cortical discontinuity and soft tissue mass with peripheral enhancement. The above features favor chondrosarcoma.

12.5 Analysis and Comments from Professor Cheng Xiao-Guang

There is high T2 signal of the lesion in the right acetabulum; however, the signal is lower when compared to the high T2 fluid signal in the urinary bladder, thus this is not a fluid-like content. Within the soft tissue mass, there is lobular morphology of high T2 signal which can be seen in chondrogenic tumor. High T2 signal can also suggest internal myxoid content. On the post-contrast images, there is typical enhancement pattern of lobular chondroid lesion, and given the patient's age and the site of involvement, this is mostly likely to be chondrosarcoma.

12.6 Diagnosis

Chondrosarcoma.

Suggested Reading

Douis H, Saifuddin A. The imaging of cartilaginous bone tumours. II. Chondrosarcoma. Skelet Radiol. 2013;42(5):611–26.

Murphey MD, Walker EA, Wilson AJ, et al. From the archives of the AFIP: imaging of primary chondrosarcoma: radiologic-pathologic correlation. Radiographics. 2003;23(5):1245–78.

Varma DG, Ayala AG, Carrasco CH, et al. Chondrosarcoma: MR imaging with pathologic correlation. Radiographics. 1992;12(4):687–704.

Ewing Sarcoma: Case 13

13

13.1 Medical History

A 7-year-old boy with left knee pain started 3 month ago without inciting event. He experienced night pain without fever. Radiograph from local hospital showed abnormality of the proximal femur, followed by open biopsy. Infectious etiology was considered, and he was treated accordingly. However, he experienced worsening symptoms after 1 month.

13.2 Physical Examination

Obvious swelling of the left proximal thigh with deformity and point tenderness. There is restricted range of motion of the left hip.

13.3 Imaging Findings

13.3.1 MR Imaging

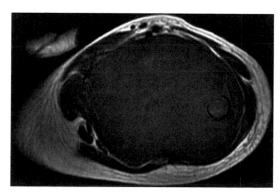

Fig. 13.1 Axial T1-weighted MR image of the left proximal femur

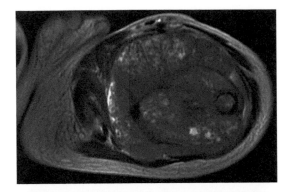

Fig. 13.2 Axial T2-weighted MR image of the left proximal femur

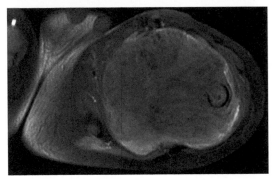

Fig. 13.3 Axial fat-suppressed post-contrast T1-weighted MR image of the left proximal femur

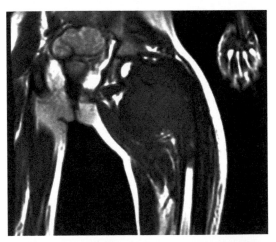

Fig. 13.4 Coronal T1-weighted MR image of the left proximal femur

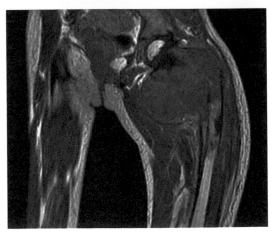

Fig. 13.5 Coronal post-contrast T1-weighted MR image of the left proximal femur

MR images of the left femur demonstrate bony destructive changes of the left proximal one third of the femur after prior open biopsy. There is an associated large soft tissue mass. There is an extensive heterogeneous enhancement.

13.4 Description and Discussion from Residents

On the MR images, there are lytic bony destructive changes of the left proximal femur with laminated periosteal reaction. There is a large soft tissue mass with internal hemorrhage of high T1 signal. No definite bone matrix is noted. There is solid enhancement. Given the patient's age and the above findings, this is likely to be Ewing sarcoma with differential diagnosis of osteosarcoma.

13.5 Analysis and Comments from Professor Cheng Xiao-Guang

MR images demonstrate left proximal femur bony destruction and large soft tissue mass. Given the patient's young age, Ewing sarcoma is at the top of the differential diagnosis. Combining radiograph, CT, and MR imaging is very important for the evaluation of bone tumor cases. Just relying on MR imaging for bone tumor evaluation would cause wrong diagnosis.

13.6 Diagnosis

Ewing sarcoma.

Suggested Reading

Murphey MD, Senchak LT, Mambalam PK, et al. From the radiologic pathology archives: Ewing sarcoma family of tumors: radiologic-pathologic correlation. Radiographics. 2013;33(3):803–31.
Wootton-Gorges SL. MR imaging of primary bone tumors and tumor-like conditions in children. Magn Reson Imaging Clin N Am. 2009;17(3):469–87.

Invasive Mesenchymal Malignant Spindle Cell Tumor: Case 14

14

14.1 Medical History

A 66-year-old female with right hip pain, swelling, and decreased range of motion for 2 months.

14.2 Physical Examination

Limping with point tenderness around the right hip and decreased range of motion.

14.3 Imaging Findings

14.3.1 Radiograph

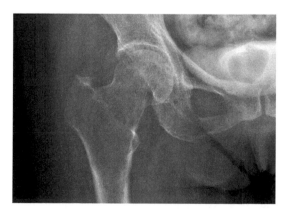

Fig. 14.1 Frontal view of the right hip

© Springer Nature Singapore Pte Ltd. and Peking Union Medical College Press 2020
X. Cheng et al., *Bone Tumor Imaging*, https://doi.org/10.1007/978-981-13-9927-5_14

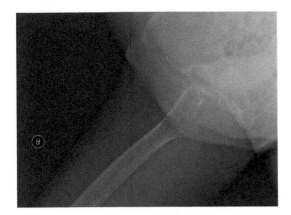

Fig. 14.2 Frog leg lateral view of the right hip

Radiographs of the right hip demonstrate lytic bony destructive changes at the right femoral neck. There is no peripheral sclerosis. There is thinning of the cortex without periosteal reaction.

14.3.2 CT Imaging

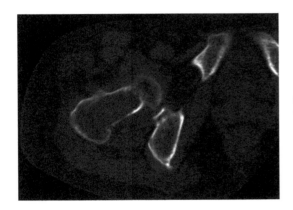

Fig. 14.3 Axial CT scan of the right hip in bone window

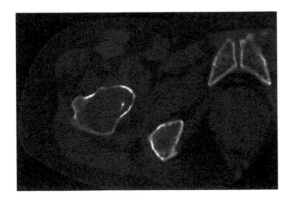

Fig. 14.4 Axial CT scan of the right hip in bone window

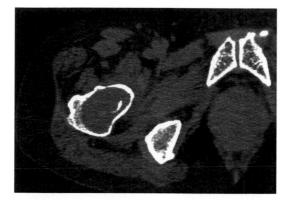

Fig. 14.5 Axial CT scan of the right hip in soft tissue window

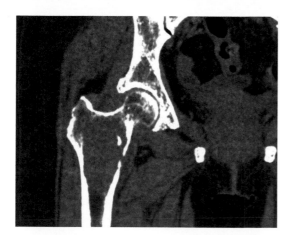

Fig. 14.6 Coronal CT scan of the right hip in soft tissue window

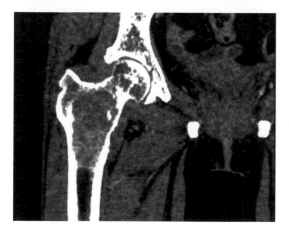

Fig. 14.7 Coronal post-contrast CT scan of the right hip in soft tissue window

CT images of the right hip demonstrate high density soft tissue lesion at the medullary cavity of the right femoral neck with clear border and internal heterogeneous densities. There are some scattered internal calcifications. There is thinning of the cortex with cortical break. There is no associated soft tissue mass or periosteal reaction. There is heterogeneous enhancement within the lesion.

14.3.3 MR Imaging

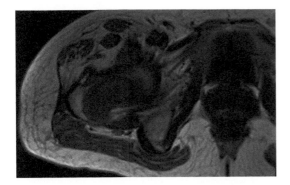

Fig. 14.8 Axial T1-weighted MR image of the right hip

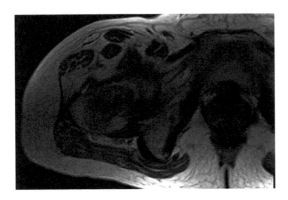

Fig. 14.9 Axial T2-weighted MR image of the right hip

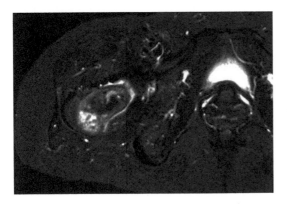

Fig. 14.10 Axial fat-suppressed T2-weighted MR image of the right hip

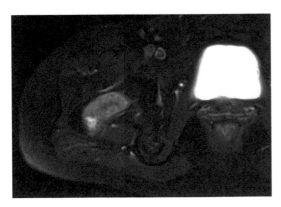

Fig. 14.11 Axial fat-suppressed post-contrast T1-weighted MR image of the right hip

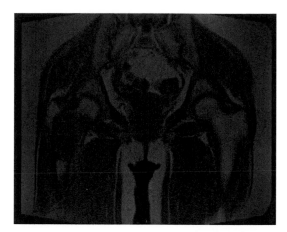

Fig. 14.12 Coronal T1-weighted MR image of the right hip

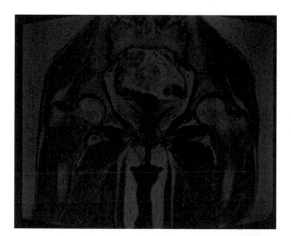

Fig. 14.13 Coronal T2-weighted MR image of the right hip

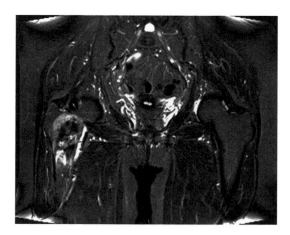

Fig. 14.14 Coronal fat-suppressed T2-weighted MR image of the right hip

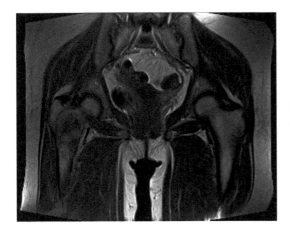

Fig. 14.15 Coronal post-contrast T1-weighted MR image of the right hip

MR images of the right hip demonstrate heterogeneous signal within the lesion at the proximal right femur. There is peripheral low T1 and high T2 signals. There is internal low T1 and low T2 signals. There is surrounding edema. There is heterogeneous enhancement within the lesion.

14.4 Description and Discussion from Residents

Radiographs of the right hip demonstrate bony destruction of the right proximal femur with ill-defined margin. There is no clear cortical break or periosteal reaction. There is no focal soft tissue mass. Given the short duration of the patient's symptoms and imaging findings, this is likely to be an aggressive lesion. There are internal heterogeneous densities on CT scan with linear and pointy calcification and cortical break and heterogeneous enhancement. Given patient's age, this is likely to be undifferentiated high-grade pleomorphic sarcoma with differential diagnosis including osteosarcoma and chondrogenic tumors. There is low T1 signal with heterogeneous T2 signal and heterogeneous enhancement on MR images. There is central region of non-enhancement. Combining CT and MR findings, undifferentiated high-grade pleomorphic sarcoma remains at the top of the differential diagnosis.

14.5 Analysis and Comments from Professor Cheng Xiao-Guang

There is a bony destruction at proximal right femur with ill-defined margin and internal heterogeneous densities/signal. There is focal pointy and linear calcification with cortical break and heterogeneous enhancement. Given the patient's age and the above imaging findings, undifferentiated high-grade pleomorphic sarcoma is at the top of the differential diagnosis. Metastatic lesion should also be included in the differential diagnosis.

14.6 Diagnosis

Invasive mesenchymal malignant spindle cell tumor.

Suggested Reading

Berner K, Johannesen TB, Hall KS, et al. Clinical epidemiology and treatment outcomes of spindle cell non-osteogenic bone sarcomas—a nationwide population-based study. J Bone Oncol. 2018;14:002–9.

Koplas MC, Lefkowitz RA, Bauer TW, et al. Imaging findings, prevalence and outcome of de novo and secondary malignant fibrous histiocytoma of bone. Skelet Radiol. 2010;39(8):791–8.

Bone Metastases: Case 15

15

15.1 Medical History

A 60-year-old male with persistent dull pain around the right hip for half a year with right lower extremity weakness and restricted activities. The patient has a history of right lesser trochanter avulsion fracture 2 years ago.

15.2 Physical Examination

No deformity noted. Mild focal point tenderness

15.3 Imaging Findings

15.3.1 Radiograph

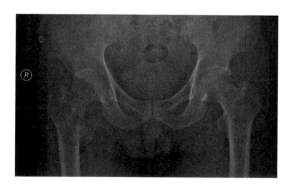

Fig. 15.1 Frontal view of the right hip

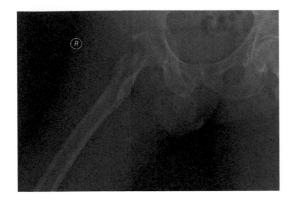

Fig. 15.2 Frog leg lateral view of the right hip

Radiographs of the right hip demonstrate lytic bony destructive changes at the right femoral head, neck, and intertrochanteric region with ill-defined border. Fragments are noted along the medial aspect of the lesser trochanter.

15.3.2 CT Imaging

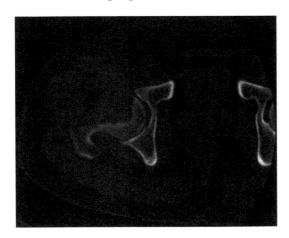

Fig. 15.3 Axial CT scan of the right hip in bone window

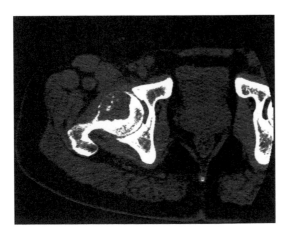

Fig. 15.4 Axial CT scan of the right hip in soft tissue window

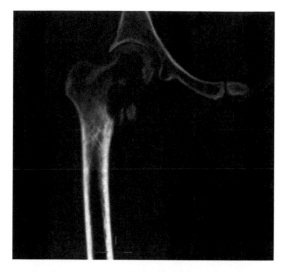

Fig. 15.5 Coronal CT scan of the right hip in bone window

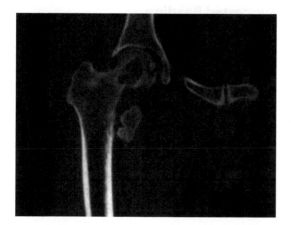

Fig. 15.6 Coronal CT scan of the right hip in bone window

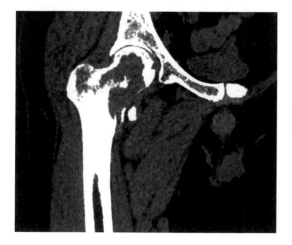

Fig. 15.7 Coronal CT scan of the right hip in soft tissue window

CT images of the right hip demonstrate multiple focal lesions with internal high densities. There is an associated soft tissue mass. Heterotopic ossifications are noted around the lesser trochanter.

15.4 Description and Discussion from Residents

Radiographs of the right hip demonstrate bony destruction of the right proximal femur with heterogeneous densities and cortical break. There is avulsion of the lesser trochanter. Malignant etiology is at the top of the differential diagnosis. Multiple focal calcifications are noted within the lytic lesion on CT scan with peripheral sclerosis and multiple areas of the involvement favor metastatic disease.

15.5 Analysis and Comments from Professor Cheng Xiao-Guang

There is a bony destruction involving right femoral head, neck, and lesser trochanter with internal heterogeneous densities and calcifications. Given the involvement of multiple regions of the proximal right femur, metastatic disease is the favored diagnosis. Differential diagnosis includes lymphoma. Lymphoma can cause multiple involvements around the medullary cavity; however, usually there is internal homogeneous densities. Bony destructive changes around the less trochanter in middle and older age patient population are usually from malignant causes and most likely from metastatic disease.

15.6 Diagnosis

Bone metastases from renal clear cell carcinoma.

Suggested Reading

Roberts CC, Daffner RH, Weissman BN, et al. ACR appropriateness criteria on metastatic bone disease. J Am Coll Radiol. 2010;7(6):400–9.
Roodman GD. Mechanisms of bone metastasis. N Engl J Med. 2004;350(16):1655–64.

16.1 Medical History

A 77-year-old female seen at outpatient clinic.

16.2 Imaging Findings

16.2.1 Radiograph

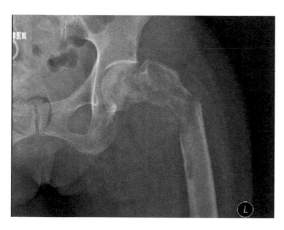

Fig. 16.1 Frontal view of the right hip

Radiograph of the left proximal femur demonstrates prominent extensive lytic bony destructive changes with cortical break. There is a suggestion of periosteal reaction with apex lateral angulation from underlying pathologic fracture. An associated soft tissue mass is noted around the bony destructive region.

16.2.2 CT Imaging

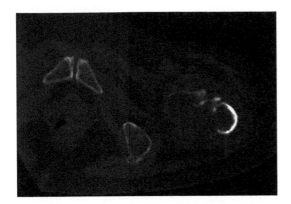

Fig. 16.2 Axial CT scan of the left proximal femur in bone window

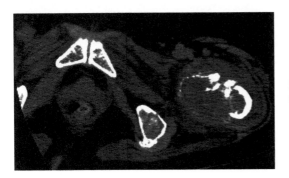

Fig. 16.3 Axial CT scan of the left proximal femur in soft tissue window

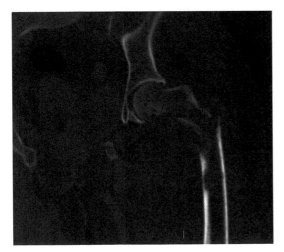

Fig. 16.4 Coronal CT scan of the left proximal femur in bone window

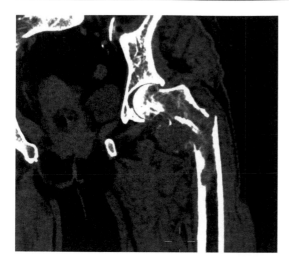

Fig. 16.5 Coronal CT scan of the left proximal femur in soft tissue window

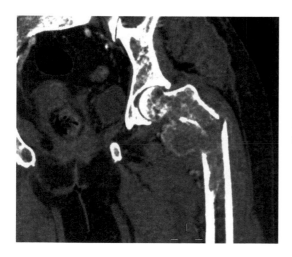

Fig. 16.6 Coronal post-contrast CT scan of the left proximal femur in soft tissue window

CT images demonstrate multiple areas of bony destruction at the left proximal femur and pelvis with focal cortical break and internal heterogeneous densities. There is a pathological fracture with apex lateral angulation. There is a soft tissue mass. Heterogeneous enhancement is also noted.

16.2.3 MR Imaging

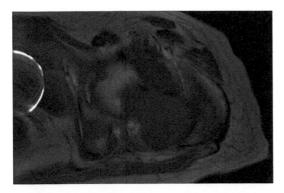

Fig. 16.7 Axial T1-weighted MR image of the left proximal femur

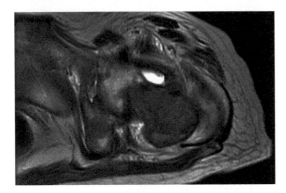

Fig. 16.8 Axial T2-weighted MR image of the left proximal femur

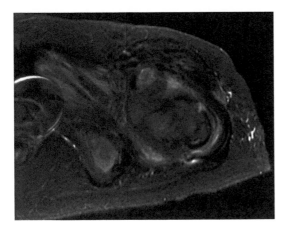

Fig. 16.9 Axial fat-suppressed T2-weighted MR image of the left proximal femur

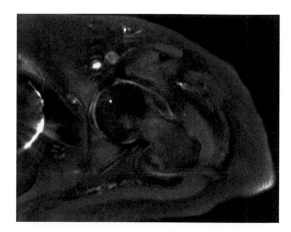

Fig. 16.10 Axial fat-suppressed post-contrast T1-weighted MR image of the left proximal femur

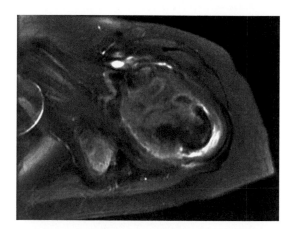

Fig. 16.11 Axial fat-suppressed post-contrast T1-weighted MR image of the left proximal femur

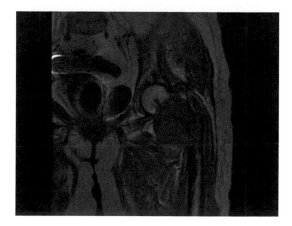

Fig. 16.12 Coronal T1-weighted MR image of the left proximal femur

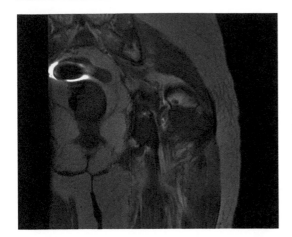

Fig. 16.13 Coronal T1-weighted MR image of the left proximal femur

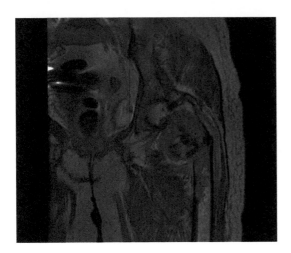

Fig. 16.14 Coronal post-contrast T1-weighted MR image of the left proximal femur

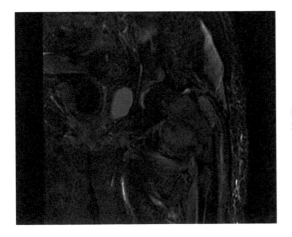

Fig. 16.15 Coronal fat-suppressed T2-weighted MR image of the left proximal femur

MR images of the left proximal femur demonstrate extensive destructive changes with low T1 signal of marrow replacement and pathological fracture. Additional lesions are noted in the left acetabulum and left pubic bone. Associated soft tissue mass is noted with extensive surrounding soft tissue edema. Heterogeneous enhancement is present.

16.3 Description and Discussion from Residents

Radiograph demonstrates ill-defined bony destruction of the left proximal femur with pathological fracture. There is an associated soft tissue mass. The above findings are consistent with malignant lesion. CT images show destruction of the proximal left femur, ilium, and pubic ramus with soft tissue mass and internal remnant of bone fragment or calcification. Given the patient's age, metastatic disease is at the top of the differential diagnosis. Lymphoma is in the differential diagnosis. MR images show multiple bone involvements with clear enhancement, consistent with metastatic disease.

16.4 Analysis and Comments from Professor Cheng Xiao-Guang

Bone destruction involving multiple bones of left femoral head and neck, lesser trochanter, acetabulum, and pubic bone with associated soft tissue mass and clear enhancement in an older patient is most suggestive of metastatic disease. Lymphoma is in the differential diagnosis.

16.5 Diagnosis

Bone metastases from breast cancer.

Suggested Reading

Liu T, Cheng T, Xu W, et al. A meta-analysis of 18FDG-PET, MRI and bone scintigraphy for diagnosis of bone metastases in patients with breast cancer. Skelet Radiol. 2011;40(5):523–31.

Roberts CC, Daffner RH, Weissman BN, et al. ACR appropriateness criteria on metastatic bone disease. J Am Coll Radiol. 2010;7(6):400–9.

Roodman GD. Mechanisms of bone metastasis. N Engl J Med. 2004;350(16):1655–64.

Lymphoma: Case 17

17

17.1 Medical History

A 28-year-old male with left hip pain and restricted activities for more than a year and limping for 4 months.

17.2 Physical Examination

Point tenderness around the left gluteal and inguinal regions. Decreased range of motion of the hip joint.

17.3 Imaging Findings

17.3.1 MR Imaging

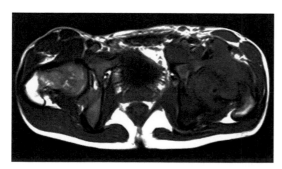

Fig. 17.1 Axial T1-weighted MR image of the left hip

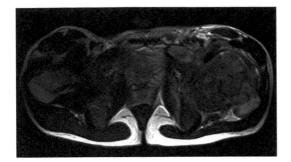

Fig. 17.2   Axial T2-weighted MR image of the left hip

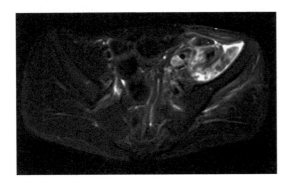

Fig. 17.3   Axial fat-suppressed T2-weighted MR image of the left hip

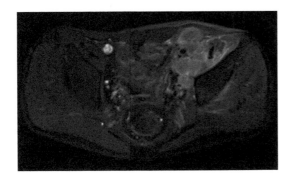

Fig. 17.4   Axial fat-suppressed post-contrast T1-weighted MR image of the left hip

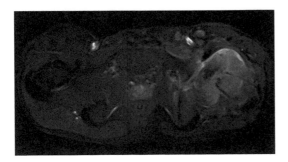

Fig. 17.5   Axial fat-suppressed post-contrast T1-weighted MR image of the left hip

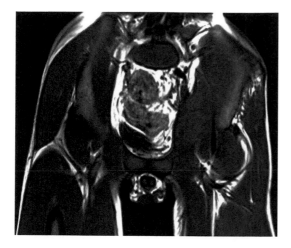

Fig. 17.6   Coronal T1-weighted MR image of the left hip

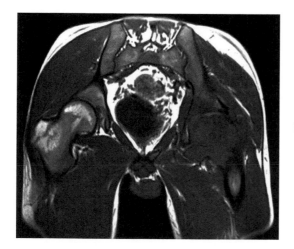

Fig. 17.7   Coronal T1-weighted MR image of the left hip

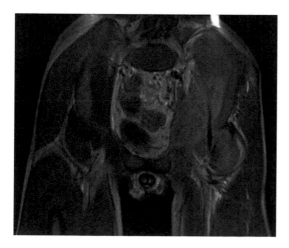

Fig. 17.8   Coronal post-contrast T1-weighted MR image of the left hip

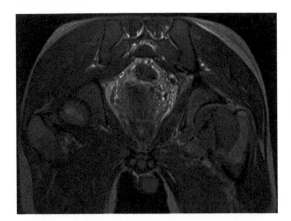

Fig. 17.9 Coronal post-contrast T1-weighted MR image of the left hip

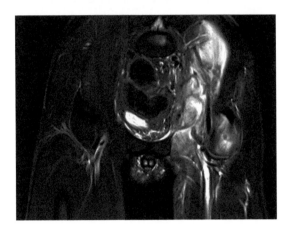

Fig. 17.10 Coronal fat-suppressed T2-weighted MR image of the left hip

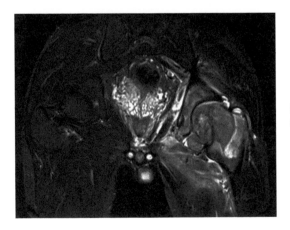

Fig. 17.11 Coronal fat-suppressed T2-weighted MR image of the left hip

MR images of the left hip demonstrate bony destruction of the left acetabulum, pubic rami, ischium, and proximal left femur with associated large soft tissue mass. There is heterogeneous signal and heterogeneous enhancement. The lesion involves the left iliopsoas and pubic musculature. Enlarged lymph nodes were noted along the left external iliac vessel and at the inguinal region.

17.4 Description and Discussion from Residents

There is an extensive abnormal signal around the left proximal femur and left iliac with surrounding soft tissue edema. Multiple foci of soft tissue abnormalities were noted in the pelvis with enhancement. Given the large area that is involved with abnormalities across a joint, infectious etiology needs to be first excluded, including tuberculosis. However, there is not much joint space narrowing, not typical of tuberculosis. There are many areas of solid soft tissue abnormalities; lymphoma should be in the differential diagnosis.

17.5 Analysis and Comments from Professor Cheng Xiao-Guang

Destruction of the femoral head with soft tissue mass extends from the cortical break with clear enhancement are not typical of tuberculosis.

Multiple soft tissue masses in the pelvis raise concern for metastatic disease. Overall, this is a malignant lesion.

17.6 Diagnosis

Lymphoma.

Suggested Reading

Hwang S. Imaging of lymphoma of the musculoskeletal system. Magn Reson Imaging Clin N Am. 2010;18(1):75–93.

Krishnan A, Shirkhoda A, Tehranzadeh J, et al. Primary bone lymphoma: radiographic-MR imaging correlation. Radiographics. 2003;23(6):1371–83.

Murphey MD, Kransdorf MJ. Primary musculoskeletal lymphoma. Radiol Clin N Am. 2016;54(4):785–95.

Weber MA, Papakonstantinou O, Nikodinovska VV, et al. Ewing's sarcoma and primary osseous lymphoma: spectrum of imaging appearances. Semin Musculoskelet Radiol. 2019;23(1):36–57.

18.1 Medical History

A 5-year-old boy with right hip pain for 8 months, with a history of fever and spontaneous resolution of the symptoms. The patient experienced another episode of right hip pain at night with night sweat about 1 month ago.

18.2 Physical Examination

Limping. The patient was not cooperative at physical exam. Point tenderness around the hip joint with warm temperature of the skin was noted compared to the contralateral side. No redness, swelling, or skin break.

18.3 Imaging Findings

18.3.1 Radiograph

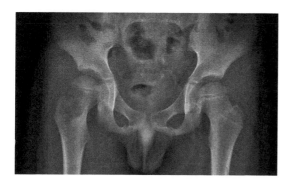

Fig. 18.1 Frontal view of the right proximal femur

© Springer Nature Singapore Pte Ltd. and Peking Union Medical College Press 2020
X. Cheng et al., *Bone Tumor Imaging*, https://doi.org/10.1007/978-981-13-9927-5_18

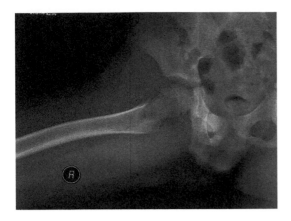

Fig. 18.2 Frog leg lateral view of the right proximal femur

Radiographs of the right hip demonstrate lytic lesion around the right femoral neck and greater trochanter with clear border and internal heterogeneous densities.

18.3.2 CT Imaging

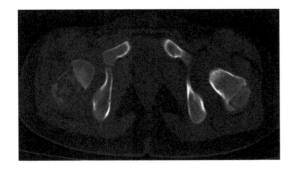

Fig. 18.3 Axial CT scan of the right proximal femur in bone window

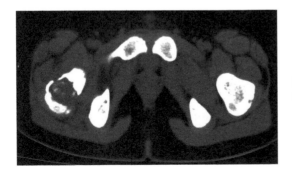

Fig. 18.4 Axial CT scan of the right proximal femur in soft tissue window

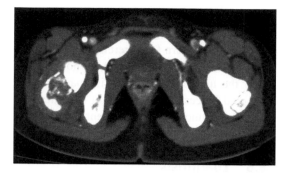

Fig. 18.5 Axial post-contrast CT scan of the right proximal femur in soft tissue window

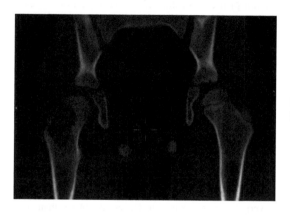

Fig. 18.6 Coronal CT scan of the right proximal femur in bone window

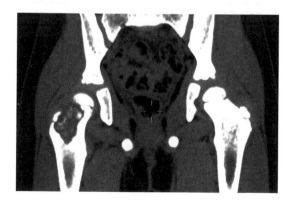

Fig. 18.7 Coronal CT scan of the right proximal femur in soft tissue window

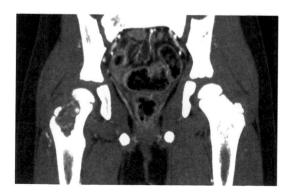

Fig. 18.8 Coronal post-contrast CT scan of the right proximal femur in soft tissue window

CT images of the right proximal femur demonstrate destructive changes, internal patchy high densities, and heterogeneous enhancement. There are multiple areas of cortical break without associated soft tissue mass.

18.4   Description and Discussion from Residents

There are lytic bony destructive changes of the right proximal femur with internal multiple patchy high densities, raising concern for sequestrum, not typical for chondral matrix. No associated soft tissue mass and heterogeneous enhancement are noted; it likely represents tuberculosis.

18.5   Analysis and Comments from Professor Cheng Xiao-Guang

A young boy with night sweats presented with lesion along the proximal femur without peripheral sclerosis but internal multiple patchy high densities, likely of sequestrum. There is a mild periosteal reaction along the cortex. Relative low density of the solid component within the lesion, though not of fluid density but with clear enhancement, raises concern for tuberculous granuloma. However, there are features that are not supportive of the tuberculosis diagnosis, mainly of no clear cold abscess in the region of bone destruction and too much solid component in the lesion.

18.6   Diagnosis

Eosinophilic granuloma (Langerhans cell histiocytosis).

Suggested Reading

Azouz EM, Saigal G, Rodriguez MM, et al. Langerhans' cell histiocytosis: pathology, imaging and treatment of skeletal involvement. Pediatr Radiol. 2005;35(2):103–15.
Samet J, Weinstein J, Fayad LM. MRI and clinical features of Langerhans cell histiocytosis (LCH) in the pelvis and extremities: can LCH really look like anything? Skelet Radiol. 2016;45(5):607–13.
Zaveri J, La Q, Yarmish G, et al. More than just Langerhans cell histiocytosis: a radiologic review of histiocytic disorders. Radiographics. 2014;34(7): 2008–24.

19.1 Medical History

A 2-year-old girl with limping on the right side for 3 months.

19.2 Physical Examination

Equal leg length of both lower extremities. No point tenderness around the hip and with normal range of motion.

19.3 Imaging Findings

19.3.1 Radiograph

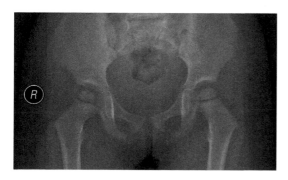

Fig. 19.1 Frontal view of the right hip

Radiograph of the right hip demonstrates focal lytic changes of the right femoral head epiphysis without peripheral sclerosis.

19.3.2 CT Imaging

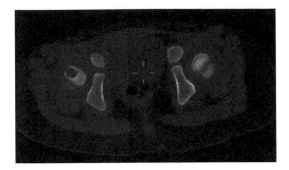

Fig. 19.2 Axial CT scan of the right hip in bone window

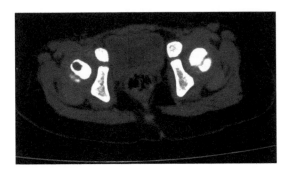

Fig. 19.3 Axial CT scan of the right hip in soft tissue window

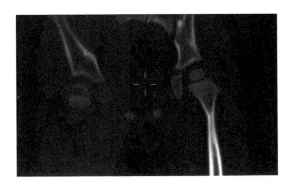

Fig. 19.4 Coronal CT scan of the right hip in bone window

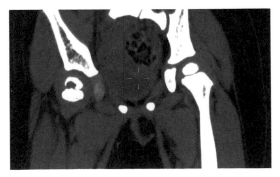

Fig. 19.5 Coronal CT scan of the right hip in soft tissue window

CT images of the right hip demonstrate the oval-shaped lytic osseous lesion in the right femoral head epiphysis with clear border. There are internal homogenous densities, mild surrounding soft tissue edema, and distention of the joint capsule.

19.3.3 MR Imaging

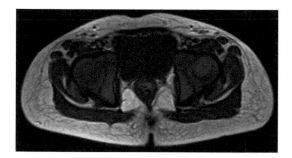

Fig. 19.6 Axial T1-weighted MR image of the right hip

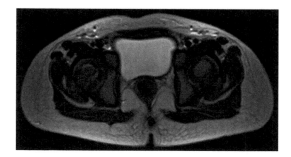

Fig. 19.7 Axial T2-weighted MR image of the right hip

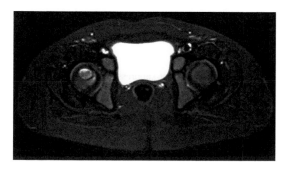

Fig. 19.8 Axial fat-suppressed T2-weighted MR image of the right hip

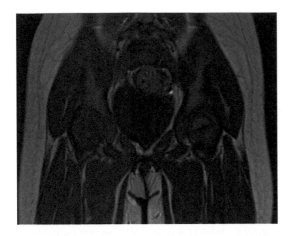

Fig. 19.9 Coronal T1-weighted MR image of the right hip

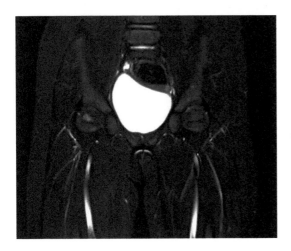

Fig. 19.10 Coronal fat-suppressed T2-weighted MR image of the right hip

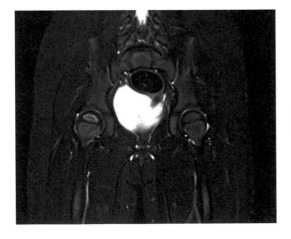

Fig. 19.11 Coronal fat-suppressed T2-weighted MR image of the right hip

MR images of the right hip demonstrate focal lesion in the right femoral head epiphysis. There is high T2 signal with adjacent marrow edema and small hip effusion.

19.4 Description and Discussion from Residents

There is lytic lesion at the right femoral head epiphysis with clear border and no internal calcification with suggestion of extension through the physis. Chondroblastoma and tuberculosis are in the differential diagnosis.

19.5 Analysis and Comments from Professor Cheng Xiao-Guang

There are reactive inflammatory changes around the lesion with internal low density and involvement of the epiphysis, tuberculosis should be excluded first, and eosinophilic granuloma should be included in the differential diagnosis. With no chondroid matrix seen on MR images and no lobulated high T2 signal and suggestion of extension through the physis, chondroblastoma can be excluded.

19.6 Diagnosis

Eosinophilic granuloma (Langerhans cell histiocytosis).

Suggested Reading

Azouz EM, Saigal G, Rodriguez MM, et al. Langerhans' cell histiocytosis: pathology, imaging and treatment of skeletal involvement. Pediatr Radiol. 2005;35(2):103–15.

Samet J, Weinstein J, Fayad LM. MRI and clinical features of Langerhans cell histiocytosis (LCH) in the pelvis and extremities: can LCH really look like anything? Skelet Radiol. 2016;45(5):607–13.

Zaveri J, La Q, Yarmish G, et al. More than just Langerhans cell histiocytosis: a radiologic review of histiocytic disorders. Radiographics. 2014;34(7):2008–24.

Tuberculosis Arthritis: Case 20

20.1   Medical History

A 7-year-old boy with left thigh kicking injury and left knee pain progressively worsening for 3 months.

20.2   Physical Examination

Forced positioning of the patient. Left hip swelling with local skin warmth and clear point tenderness.

20.3   Imaging Findings

20.3.1 Radiograph

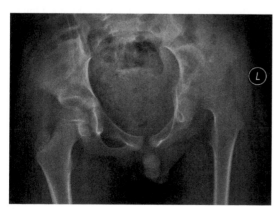

Fig. 20.1 Frontal view of the left hip

Radiograph of the left hip shows decreased bone density around the left hip with irregular joint space and narrowing. There is superior migration of the left proximal femur with varus angulation and joint swelling.

20.3.2 CT Imaging

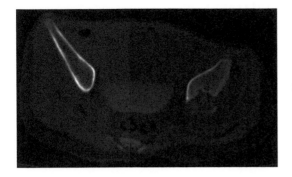

Fig. 20.2 Axial CT scan of the left hip in bone window

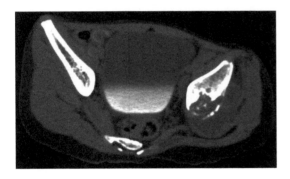

Fig. 20.3 Axial CT scan of the left hip in soft tissue window

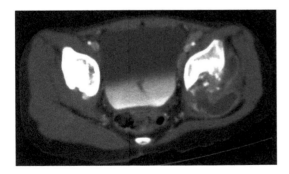

Fig. 20.4 Axial post-contrast CT scan of the left hip in soft tissue window

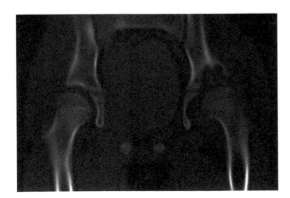

Fig. 20.5 Coronal CT scan of the left hip in bone window

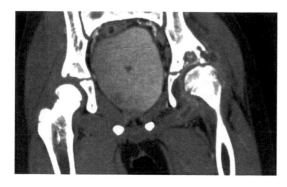

Fig. 20.6 Coronal post-contrast CT scan of the left hip in soft tissue window

CT scan of the left hip demonstrates multiple areas of destruction around the left acetabulum with internal high densities. There is joint effusion with synovial hyperplasia and enhancement.

20.3.3 MR Imaging

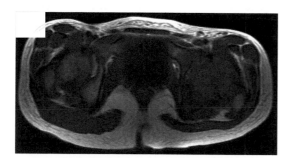

Fig. 20.7 Axial T1-weighted MR image of the left hip

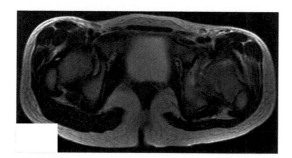

Fig. 20.8 Axial T2-weighted MR image of the left hip

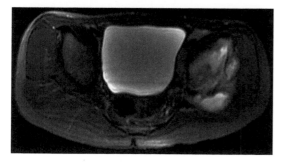

Fig. 20.9 Axial fat-suppressed T2-weighted MR image of the left hip

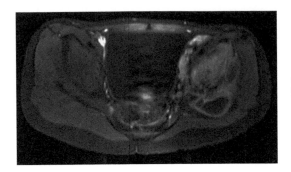

Fig. 20.10 Axial post-contrast fat-suppressed T1-weighted MR image of the left hip

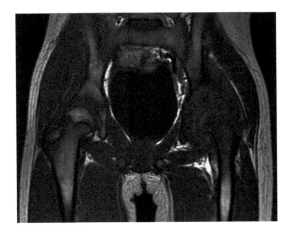

Fig. 20.11 Coronal T1-weighted MR image of the left hip

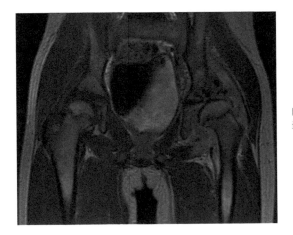

Fig. 20.12 Coronal post-contrast T1-weighted MR image of the left hip

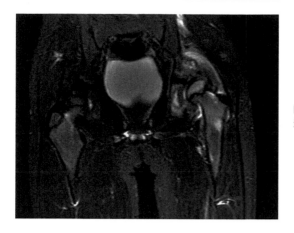

Fig. 20.13 Coronal fat-suppressed T2-weighted MR image of the left hip

MR images of the left hip demonstrate bony destruction around the left hip. There is destruction of the articular cartilage with marrow edema across the left hip joint. Left hip joint effusion, synovial hyperplasia, and surrounding soft tissue edema are noted with enhancement.

20.4 Description and Discussion from Residents

Radiograph of a 7-year-old boy demonstrates left hip subluxation with irregular left acetabulum and decreased bone densities around left proximal femur indicating osteopenia. Multiple foci of bone destruction of the left acetabulum with internal calcifications and bone fragments with periosteal reaction and irregular shape of the epiphysis are noted on CT scan. There is also soft tissue swelling with multiloculated peripherally enhancing fluid collection. Similar findings are noted on MR images with marrow edema across the left hip, most indicative of infection, likely tuberculosis.

20.5 Analysis and Comments from Professor Cheng Xiao-Guang

Radiograph demonstrates forced position of the patient with pelvic tilt and left hip subluxation with periarticular osteopenia. Left acetabular bone destruction with bone fragments and peri-

osteal reaction, and irregular shape of the femoral head are noted on bone windows of the CT scan. Extensive soft tissue swelling with abscess and joint effusion are noted on soft tissue windows of the CT scan. Peripherally enhancing fluid collection with changeable morphology and location likely represents "cold abscess," indicative of tuberculosis arthritis. Proximal femur abnormalities with edema and articular surface, cartilage irregularities, and abscess are all indicative of infection, favoring tuberculosis arthritis. Differential diagnosis: (1) bacterial septic arthritis: usually the patient presents with fast clinical course with serious symptoms and elevated white count, usually no "sand-like" bone fragments on imaging; (2) chondroblastoma: it could affect acetabulum or femoral head with surrounding reactive changes, but no abnormalities across the joint; (3) eosinophilic granuloma: again it would not cause abnormalities across the joint.

20.6 Diagnosis

Tuberculosis arthritis.

Suggested Reading

De Backer AI, Mortelé KJ, Vanhoenacker FM, et al. Imaging of extraspinal musculoskeletal tuberculosis. Eur J Radiol. 2006;57(1):119–30.
Prasad A, Manchanda S, Sachdev N, et al. Imaging features of pediatric musculoskeletal tuberculosis. Pediatr Radiol. 2012;42(10):1235–49.

21.1 Medical History

A 46-year-old male was seen at the outpatient clinic for 4-month follow-up of left lower extremity fracture.

21.2 Imaging Findings

21.2.1 CT Imaging

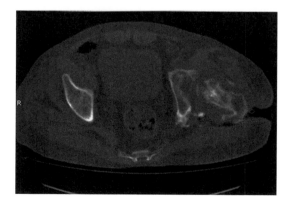

Fig. 21.1 Axial CT scan of the left hip in bone window

© Springer Nature Singapore Pte Ltd. and Peking Union Medical College Press 2020
X. Cheng et al., *Bone Tumor Imaging*, https://doi.org/10.1007/978-981-13-9927-5_21

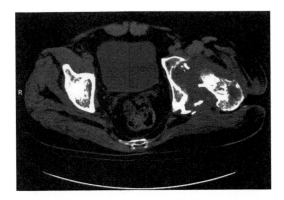

Fig. 21.2 Axial CT scan of the left hip in soft tissue window

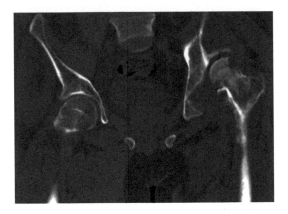

Fig. 21.3 Coronal CT scan of the left hip in bone window

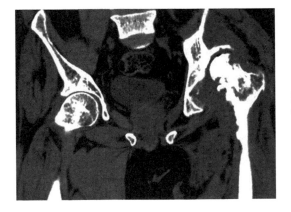

Fig. 21.4 Coronal CT scan of the left hip in soft tissue window

CT images of the left hip demonstrate bony destruction around the left hip with periarticular osteopenia. There are internal high densities. Joint effusion and adjacent soft tissue edema are noted. There is superior migration of the proximal femur with varus angulation.

21.3 Description and Discussion from Residents

Subluxation of the left hip with superior migration of the proximal left femur with varus angulation is noted in a middle-aged male patient with a history of surgery. There is clear destruction of the proximal femur with internal multiple foci of high densities likely sequestrum and suggestion of sinus track formation, infection is at the top of the differential diagnosis. Bacterial septic arthritis and chronic osteomyelitis are all in the differential diagnosis including tuberculosis. Periarticular osteopenia is noted, but this could be caused by disuse, not necessarily related to underlying condition.

21.4 Analysis and Comments from Professor Cheng Xiao-Guang

Imaging findings of subluxation of the left femoral head with destruction and joint effusion and internal high densities and suggestion of sinus tract are most consistent with infection, favoring bacterial septic arthritis. If there is prolonged clinical history, then tuberculosis should be included in the differential diagnosis. Combining clinical history with laboratory tests is essential for making the final diagnosis.

21.5 Diagnosis

Septic arthritis (drug-resistant *Staphylococcus aureus*).

Suggested Reading

Beaman FD, von Herrmann PF, Kransdorf MJ, et al. ACR appropriateness criteria® suspected osteomyelitis, septic arthritis, or soft tissue infection (excluding spine and diabetic foot). J Am Coll Radiol. 2017;14(5S):S326–37.

Rupasov A, Cain U, Montoya S, et al. Imaging of post-traumatic arthritis, avascular necrosis, septic arthritis, complex regional pain syndrome, and cancer mimicking arthritis. Radiol Clin N Am. 2017;55(5):1111–30.

22.1   Medical History

A 32-year-old female seen at an outpatient clinic.

22.2   Imaging Findings

22.2.1 Radiograph

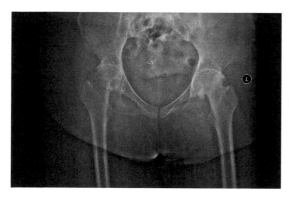

Fig. 22.1 Frontal view of the pelvis

Radiograph of the pelvis demonstrates decreased bone densities around both hips. There are arthritic changes of both hips as osteophytes formation with joint space narrowing and subchondral sclerosis, unusual for the patient's age.

© Springer Nature Singapore Pte Ltd. and Peking Union Medical College Press 2020
X. Cheng et al., *Bone Tumor Imaging*, https://doi.org/10.1007/978-981-13-9927-5_22

22.2.2 CT Imaging

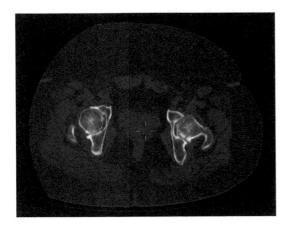

Fig. 22.2 Axial CT scan of both hips in bone window

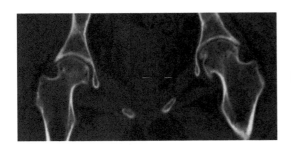

Fig. 22.3 Coronal CT scan of both hips in bone window

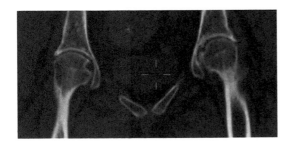

Fig. 22.4 Coronal CT scan of both hips in bone window

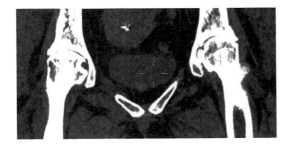

Fig. 22.5 Coronal CT scan of both hips in soft tissue window

CT scan of the hips demonstrates bilateral axial joint space narrowing of the hips. There are osteophytes formation. No joint effusion is noted.

22.3 Description and Discussion from Residents

There are arthritic changes of both hips with osteophytes formation, subchondral sclerosis, joint space loss, and decreased bone densities. The above findings are uncommon for the patient's age and raise concern for underlying inflammatory condition, such as rheumatoid arthritis.

22.4 Analysis and Comments from Professor Cheng Xiao-Guang

Osteophyte formation with subchondral sclerosis is consistent with imaging findings of osteoarthritis. However, this is very uncommon for the patient's young age. Additionally, there are decreased bone densities around the joints with axial joint space narrowing, not usually seen with osteoarthritis. Clinical correlation is needed for final diagnosis.

22.5 Diagnosis

Rheumatoid arthritis.

Suggested Reading

Barile A, Arrigoni F, Bruno F, et al. Computed tomography and MR imaging in rheumatoid arthritis. Radiol Clin N Am. 2017;55(5):997–1007.

Llopis E, Kroon HM, Acosta J. Conventional radiology in rheumatoid arthritis. Radiol Clin N Am. 2017;55(5):917–41.

Sommer OJ, Kladosek A, Weiler V, et al. Rheumatoid arthritis: a practical guide to state-of-the-art imaging, image interpretation, and clinical implications. Radiographics. 2005;25(2):381–98.

Rheumatoid Arthritis: Case 23

23

23.1 Medical History

A 49-year-old male with left hip pain for 10 years and worsening decreased activities for 2 years.

23.2 Physical Examination

Both hips demonstrated shortening with flexion deformities and markedly decreased range of motion.

23.3 Imaging Findings

23.3.1 Radiograph

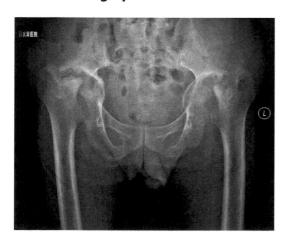

Fig. 23.1 Frontal view of the pelvis

© Springer Nature Singapore Pte Ltd. and Peking Union Medical College Press 2020
X. Cheng et al., *Bone Tumor Imaging*, https://doi.org/10.1007/978-981-13-9927-5_23

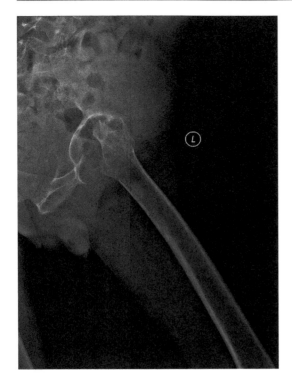

Fig. 23.2 Frog leg lateral view of the left hip

Radiographs of the hips demonstrate bilateral proximal femur destruction with absorption and non-visualization of the femoral heads. Secondary deepening of the acetabula bilaterally is noted. There are decreased bone densities around the hips.

23.3.2 CT Imaging

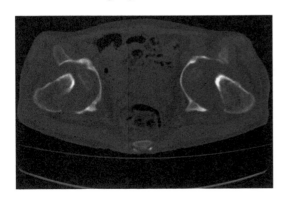

Fig. 23.3 Axial CT scan of both hips in bone window

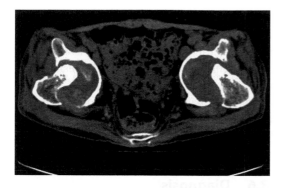

Fig. 23.4 Axial CT scan of both hips in soft tissue window

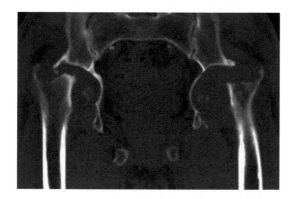

Fig. 23.5 Coronal CT scan of both hips in bone window

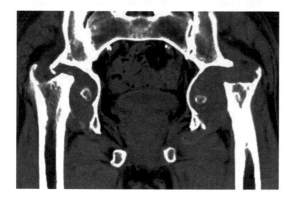

Fig. 23.6 Coronal CT scan of both hips in soft tissue window

CT images of the hips demonstrate marked destruction of proximal femurs involving the bilateral femoral heads and necks. There are absorption, fragmentation, and deformities. There are secondary irregularities along the articular surface with enlargement of the joint capsules. Osteophytes are noted. Superior migration of the proximal femur is noted with varus angulation. Remodeling of the acetabula are noted bilaterally with deepening and enlargement, suggesting chronicity of the condition.

23.4   Description and Discussion from Residents

Radiographs show bilateral relatively symmetric destruction with non-visualization of the femoral heads and necks and superior migration of the femur with varus angulation and deepening of the acetabula and osteophytes formation with subchondral sclerosis in a middle-aged man with chronic clinical course. Bilateral hip joint effusions with internal multiple high densities of calcifications or bone fragments within the destruction are noted on CT scan. The joint effusion does not appear complex. Underlying inflammatory condition is at the top of the differential diagnosis. Symmetric joint distribution is suggestive of rheumatoid arthritis. However, middle-aged man is not the typical population to be affected by rheumatoid arthritis. Differential diagnosis includes tuberculosis, given the chronic course, though symmetric involvement is rare in tuberculosis.

23.5   Analysis and Comments from Professor Cheng Xiao-Guang

Bilateral femoral head and neck destruction with fragments inferiorly are noted on radiographs with clear decreased bone densities around the joints.

There is irregular right sacroiliac joint with relatively normal left sacroiliac joint. Residual proximal bilateral femurs show sclerosis at the tip on CT scan with joint effusion and high densities. The patient complains of pain, excluding the possibilities of neuropathic joint. This could represent rheumatoid arthritis; however, such extensive bone destruction is uncommon in rheumatoid arthritis.

23.6   Diagnosis

Rheumatoid arthritis.

Suggested Reading

Barile A, Arrigoni F, Bruno F, et al. Computed tomography and MR imaging in rheumatoid arthritis. Radiol Clin N Am. 2017;55(5):997–1007.

Llopis E, Kroon HM, Acosta J. Conventional radiology in rheumatoid arthritis. Radiol Clin N Am. 2017;55(5):917–41.

Sommer OJ, Kladosek A, Weiler V, et al. Rheumatoid arthritis: a practical guide to state-of-the-art imaging, image interpretation, and clinical implications. Radiographics. 2005;25(2):381–98.

24.1 Medical History

A 29-year-old male with pain and swelling around multiple joints for 7 years and worsening for about a month.

24.2 Physical Examination

Swelling and point tenderness around multiple joints with decreased range of motion.

24.3 Imaging Findings

24.3.1 Radiograph

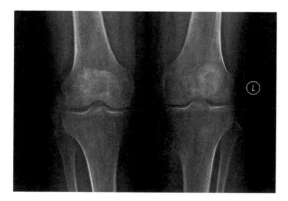

Fig. 24.1 Frontal view of both knees

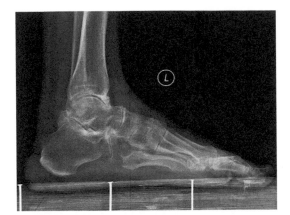

Fig. 24.2 Lateral view of the left ankle and foot

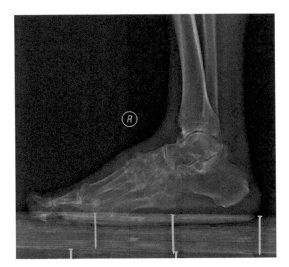

Fig. 24.3 Lateral view of the right ankle and foot

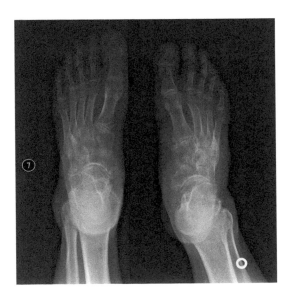

Fig. 24.4 Frontal view of both feet

Radiographs of knees and feet demonstrate multiple soft tissue nodules around the joints, such as lateral aspect of the right knee, medial aspect of the left proximal tibia, dorsal aspect of the left talonavicular joint and heel, and dorsal over the right midfoot.

24.3.2 CT Imaging

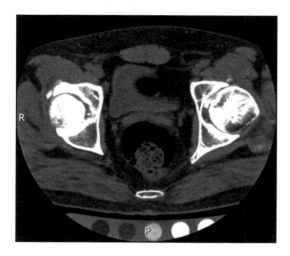

Fig. 24.5 Axial CT scan of both hips in soft tissue window

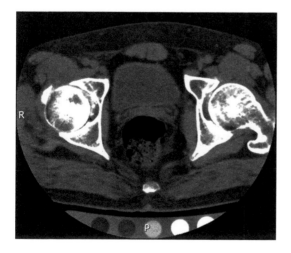

Fig. 24.6 Axial CT scan of both hips in soft tissue window

CT images of the hips demonstrate several patchy densities within both hip joints.

24.4　Description and Discussion from Residents

Mild decreased bone densities around both knees, ankles, and feet with soft tissue swelling and multiple soft tissue high densities around both hips, lateral aspect of the right knee, medial aspect of the left knee, and dorsal aspect of the left foot and heel are noted. Focal erosions around the left first metatarsal head and both naviculars with surrounding soft tissue swelling are also present. The above combinations of findings in a young male with chronic disease course are most suggestive of gouty arthritis.

24.5　Analysis and Comments from Professor Cheng Xiao-Guang

Correlation with clinical history is very important for radiologists to diagnose inflammatory arthropathy. This patient's images demonstrate decreased bone densities around both knees, ankles, and feet, soft tissue nodule around the knee with high density, increased density around Hoffa's fat pad, osteophyte formation around ankle joints, soft tissue swelling, erosion at distal left first metatarsal, and high densities in both hip joints. In a young male patient with multiple joint involvements, gouty arthritis is at the top of the differential diagnosis. However, the typical erosion at the first metatarsal is not obvious; correlation with uric acid level is recommended.

24.6　Diagnosis

Gouty arthritis.

Suggested Reading

Buckens CF, Terra MP, Maas M. Computed tomography and MR imaging in crystalline-induced Arthropathies. Radiol Clin N Am. 2017;55(5):1023–34.
Omoumi P, Zufferey P, Malghem J, et al. Imaging in gout and other crystal-related Arthropathies. Rheum Dis Clin N Am. 2016;42(4):621–44.

Septic Arthritis: Case 25

25

25.1   Medical History

A 75-year-old male with draining and nonhealing ulcer of the right heel for 6 months now presents with left hip pain and restricted activities.

25.2   Physical Examination

Left hip swelling and point tenderness

25.3   Imaging Findings

25.3.1 Radiograph

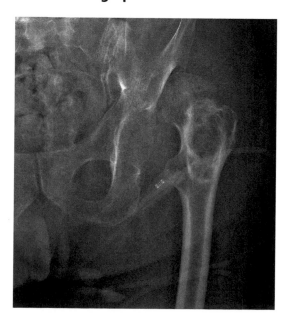

Fig. 25.1 Frontal view of the left hip

Radiograph of the left hip demonstrates bone destruction of left proximal femur with peripheral sclerosis and superior migration of the left femoral head and surrounding soft tissue swelling.

25.3.2 CT Imaging

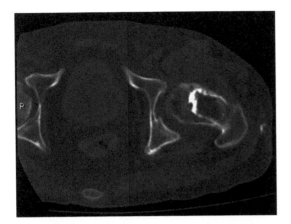

Fig. 25.2 Axial CT scan of the left hip in bone window

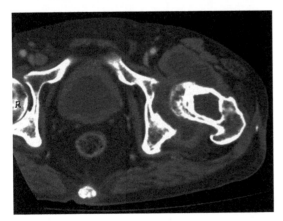

Fig. 25.3 Axial post-contrast CT scan of the left hip in soft tissue window

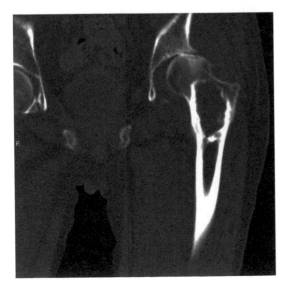

Fig. 25.4 Coronal CT scan of the left hip in bone window

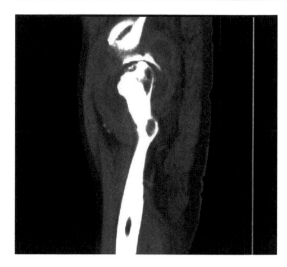

Fig. 25.5 Sagittal post-contrast CT scan of the left hip in soft tissue window

CT images of the left hip demonstrate geographic lytic bone destruction at left femoral neck and intertrochanteric region with clear border, sclerosis, and joint effusion. There is a peripheral thick-walled enhancement of the joint capsule. There is also subluxation of the left hip.

25.3.3 MR Imaging

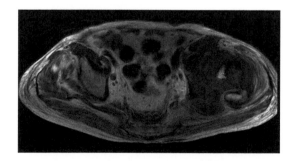

Fig. 25.6 Axial T1-weighted MR image of the left hip

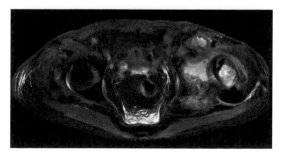

Fig. 25.7 Axial fat-suppressed T2-weighted MR image of the left hip

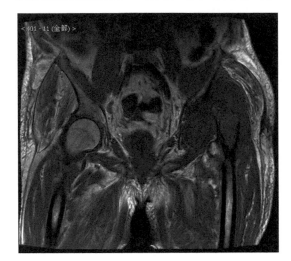

Fig. 25.8 Coronal T1-weighted MR image of the left hip

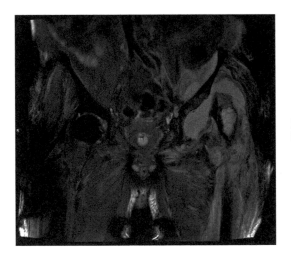

Fig. 25.9 Coronal fat-suppressed T2-weighted MR image of the left hip

MR images of the left hip demonstrate abnormalities of the left femoral neck and intertrochanteric region with low T1 and high T2 signal. There is synovial hyperplasia with effusion and atrophy of the surrounding soft tissue with edema. Similar low T1 and high T2 signals are also noted along the left acetabulum with subluxation of the left hip joint.

25.4 Description and Discussion from Residents

The imaging features of the case are bone destruction at the left intertrochanteric region with peripheral sclerosis, internal homogenous densities, destruction at the femoral head, synovial hyperplasia with joint effusion, internal multiple foci of sandy-like high densities, subluxation of the left hip with superior and lateral translation of the femoral head, adjacent soft tissue edema, and peripheral thick-walled enhancement. Combining the above imaging features with clinical history of draining foot ulcer, bacterial septic joint is the most likely diagnosis; however, tuberculosis cannot be excluded.

25.5 Analysis and Comments from Professor Cheng Xiao-Guang

The patient presented with clinical history of draining ulcer. Left intertrochanteric bone destruction with sclerosis and femoral head destruction with adjacent multiple high densities with large joint effusion are noted on imaging. Thick-walled peripheral enhancement is noted on the post-contrast CT scan, representing abscess. History of heel draining ulcer raises concern for hematogenous spread of infection. Extensive surrounding soft tissue edema seen on MR also reflects inflammation. Further investigation with laboratory tests to differentiate bacterial septic arthritis from tuberculosis is recommended. The absence of clear periarticular osteopenia on imaging is not supportive of tuberculosis.

25.6 Diagnosis

Septic arthritis (*Staphylococcus aureus*).

Suggested Reading

Beaman FD, von Herrmann PF, Kransdorf MJ, et al. ACR appropriateness criteria® suspected osteomyelitis, septic arthritis, or soft tissue infection (excluding spine and diabetic foot). J Am Coll Radiol. 2017;14(5S):S326–37.

Rupasov A, Cain U, Montoya S, et al. Imaging of post-traumatic arthritis, avascular necrosis, septic arthritis, complex regional pain syndrome, and cancer mimicking arthritis. Radiol Clin N Am. 2017;55(5):1111–30.

26.1 Medical History

A 29-year-old male with left knee pain for 5 months and worsening with restricted activities for 8 days.

26.2 Physical Examination

Point tenderness with decreased range of motion.

26.3 Imaging Findings

26.3.1 Radiograph

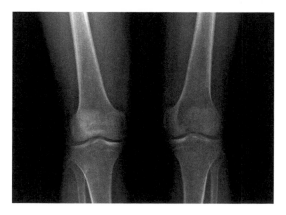

Fig. 26.1 Frontal view of the left knee

© Springer Nature Singapore Pte Ltd. and Peking Union Medical College Press 2020
X. Cheng et al., *Bone Tumor Imaging*, https://doi.org/10.1007/978-981-13-9927-5_26

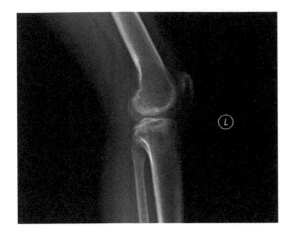

Fig. 26.2 Lateral view of the left knee

Radiographs of the left knee demonstrate a well-defined low-density lesion at the distal left femur. There is no peripheral sclerosis or periosteal reaction. There is soft tissue density along the posterior distal femur on the lateral view.

26.3.2 CT Imaging

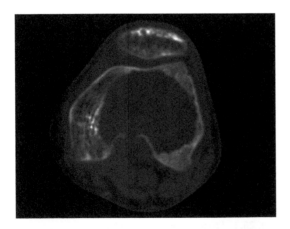

Fig. 26.3 Axial CT scan of the left knee in bone window

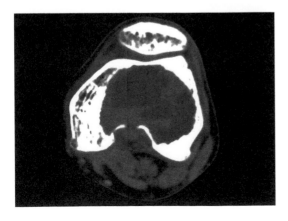

Fig. 26.4 Axial CT scan of the left knee in soft tissue window

CT images of the left knee demonstrate well-defined, irregular border of the lytic lesion at the distal femur. There is posterior cortical break with soft tissue mass that extends beyond the break. Internal heterogeneous densities are noted with septations and fluid-fluid levels.

26.3.3 MR Imaging

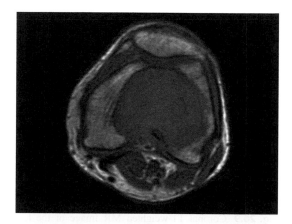

Fig. 26.5 Axial T1-weighted MR image of the left knee

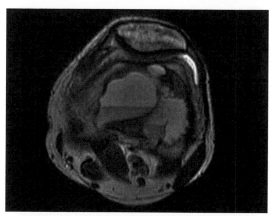

Fig. 26.6 Axial T2-weighted MR image of the left knee

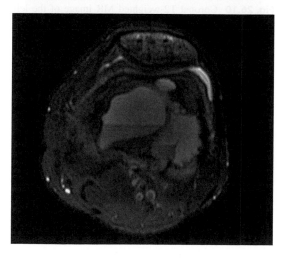

Fig. 26.7 Axial fat-suppressed T2-weighted MR image of the left knee

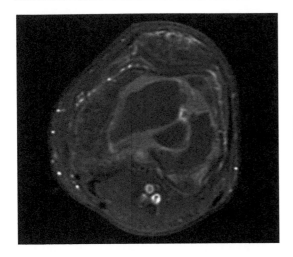

Fig. 26.8 Axial post-contrast fat-suppressed T1-weighted MR image of the left knee

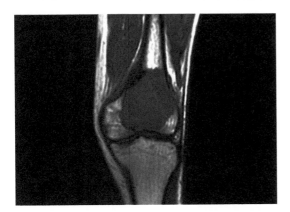

Fig. 26.9 Coronal T1-weighted MR image of the left knee

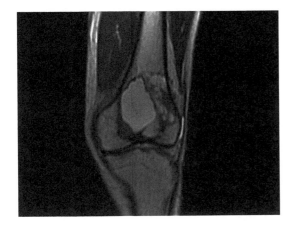

Fig. 26.10 Coronal T2-weighted MR image of the left knee

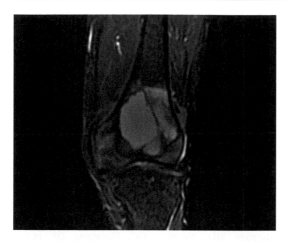

Fig. 26.11 Coronal fat-suppressed T2-weighted MR image of the left knee

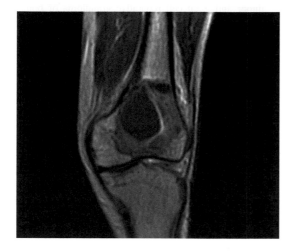

Fig. 26.12 Coronal post-contrast T1-weighted MR image of the left knee

MR images of the left knee demonstrate the lesion in the left distal femur with internal heterogeneous signal, predominantly of low T1 and heterogeneous high T2 signals. There are internal septations with multiple fluid-fluid levels and enhancement of the septations.

26.4   Description and Discussion from Residents

The patient is a young male. Radiographs demonstrate lytic lesion of the left distal femur with clear border, suggesting peripheral sclerosis and no definite cortical break. On CT scan, there is a slightly expansile distal femoral lesion with thinning of the posterior cortex and soft tissue mass extending from the focal cortical break and internal heterogeneous densities with fluid-fluid levels and no calcification. Given the patient's age, clinical history, and location of the lesion, the most likely diagnosis is giant cell tumor with secondary aneurysmal bone cyst (ABC); however, secondary ABC from malignant lesion or telangiectatic osteosarcoma needs to be excluded. On MR imaging, there are cystic and solid components of the lesion with heterogeneous signal and soft tissue mass but no significant surrounding marrow edema, consistent with giant cell tumor with secondary ABC.

26.5   Analysis and Comments from Professor Cheng Xiao-Guang

The patient presented with a slightly expansile distal femoral lesion with well-defined border and associated soft tissue mass. CT scan demonstrates internal cystic component. Fluid-fluid levels and enhancement of the solid components are demonstrated on MRI. In an adult male patient, all the above imaging findings support the diagnosis of giant cell tumor. There is a small amount of soft tissue mass extending beyond the cortex; however, combining CT and MR images, giant cell tumor with secondary ABC is at the top of the differential diagnosis. Some radiologists suggested to exclude telangiectatic osteosarcoma, for that there is usually more solid enhancing component with less cystic septations, thus unlikely for the current case. Giant cell tumor is the most common enhancing epiphyseal lesion, followed by vascular lesion.

26.6   Diagnosis

Giant cell tumor of bone with secondary ABC.

Suggested Reading

Aoki J, Tanikawa H, Ishii K, et al. MR findings indicative of hemosiderin in giant-cell tumor of bone: frequency, cause, and diagnostic significance. AJR Am J Roentgenol. 1996;166(1):145–8.

Chakarun CJ, Forrester DM, Gottsegen CJ, et al. Giant cell tumor of bone: review, mimics, and new developments in treatment. Radiographics. 2013;33(1):197–211.

Murphey MD, Nomikos GC, Flemming DJ, et al. From the archives of AFIP. Imaging of giant cell tumor and giant cell reparative granuloma of bone: radiologic-pathologic correlation. Radiographics. 2001;21(5):1283–309.

27.1 Medical History

A 41-year-old female with mass seen on left distal thigh. MRI performed for injury about 3 month ago. No complaints of pain.

27.2 Physical Examination

Mass around the posterior and medial aspect of the left thigh, solid with clear border, smooth, and movable.

27.3 Imaging Findings

27.3.1 Radiograph

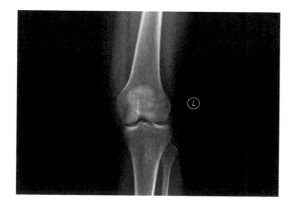

Fig. 27.1 Frontal view of the left knee

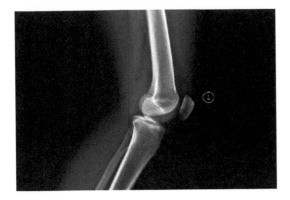

Fig. 27.2 Lateral view of the left knee

Radiographs of the left knee demonstrate a soft tissue lesion along the left medial femoral condyle on the frontal view and posterior on the lateral view. There is a clear border of the lesion with homogeneous densities.

27.3.2 CT Imaging

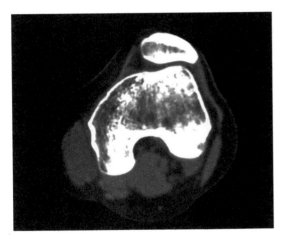

Fig. 27.3 Axial CT scan of the left knee in soft tissue window

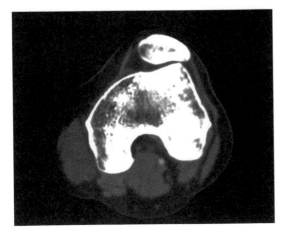

Fig. 27.4 Axial post-contrast CT scan of the left knee in soft tissue window

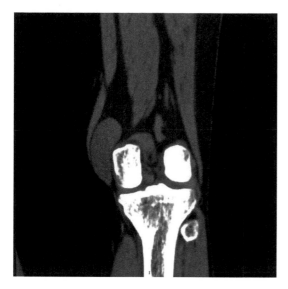

Fig. 27.5 Coronal CT scan of the left knee in soft tissue window

CT images of the left knee demonstrate a well-defined soft tissue mass along the medial distal femoral condyle and extending posteriorly. No clear enhancement is noted.

27.3.3 MR Imaging

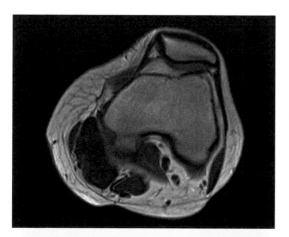

Fig. 27.6 Axial T1-weighted MR image of the left knee

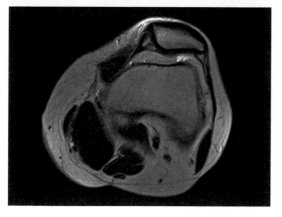

Fig. 27.7 Axial T2-weighted MR image of the left knee

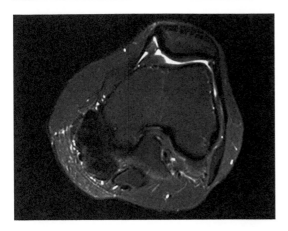

Fig. 27.8 Axial fat-suppressed T2-weighted MR image of the left knee

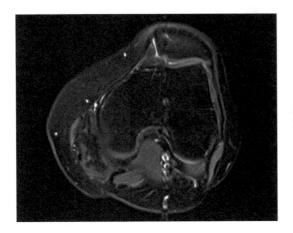

Fig. 27.9 Axial post-contrast fat-suppressed T1-weighted MR image of the left knee

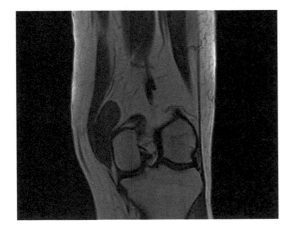

Fig. 27.10 Coronal T1-weighted MR image of the left knee

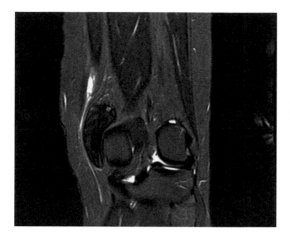

Fig. 27.11 Coronal fat-suppressed T2-weighted MR image of the left knee

MR images of the left knee demonstrate the multiple linear signals within the soft tissue lesion. Mild enhancement is noted peripherally. There is no invasion to the underlying osseous structures. No marrow edema is noted.

27.4 Description and Discussion from Residents

The patient is a female. Radiographs demonstrate soft tissue lesion along the medial femoral condyle with clear border and no invasion to the bone. On CT scan, the lesion demonstrates similar density as the muscle without bone invasion or periosteal reaction. There is less enhancement of the lesion compared to adjacent muscles. This is likely a benign lesion, given the clinical course and imaging findings. Differential diagnoses include hematoma, myositis ossificans, and tenosynovial giant cell tumor. There is low T1 and low T2 signals, suggesting internal hemosiderin, and no adjacent marrow edema and no obvious enhancement on MR images, likely representing tenosynovial giant cell tumor.

27.5 Analysis and Comments from Professor Cheng Xiao-Guang

The patient is a female. Radiographs demonstrate soft tissue mass along the medial femoral condyle with clear border and no bone invasion. CT scan demonstrates mass at posterior knee adjacent to the muscle with no clear enhancement; synovial sarcoma cannot be excluded. The lesion demonstrates low signals on T1, T2, and fat-suppressed sequences with suggestion of internal hemosiderin, raises concern for tenosynovial giant cell tumor vs. synovial sarcoma. Imaging findings do not support the diagnose of hematoma.

27.6 Diagnosis

Fibroma of tendon sheath.

Suggested Reading

Ge Y, Guo, You Y, et al. Magnetic resonance imaging features of fibromas and giant cell tumors of the tendon sheath: differential diagnosis. Eur Radiol. 2019;29(7):3441–9. https://doi.org/10.1007/s00330-019-06226-4.

Suzuki K, Yasuda T, Suzawa S, et al. Fibroma of tendon sheath around large joints: clinical characteristics and literature review. BMC Musculoskelet Disord. 2017;18(1):376.

28.1 Medical History

A 12-year-old boy presented with left femur swelling and pain, worsening at night, 4 months after fall.

28.2 Physical Examination

Flexion deformity of the left knee with muscle atrophy.

28.3 Imaging Findings

28.3.1 Radiograph

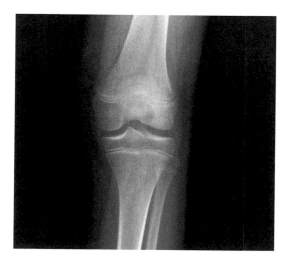

Fig. 28.1 Frontal view of the left knee

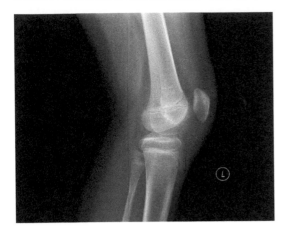

Fig. 28.2 Lateral view of the left knee

Radiographs of the left knee demonstrate an oval region of low density at the distal femoral epiphysis with clear border, peripheral sclerosis, internal heterogeneous density, and no cortical break.

28.3.2 CT Imaging

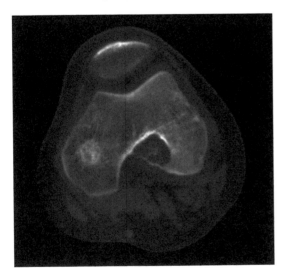

Fig. 28.3 Axial CT scan of the left knee in bone window

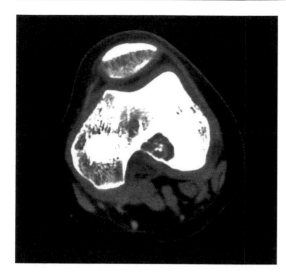

Fig. 28.4 Axial CT scan of the left knee in soft tissue window

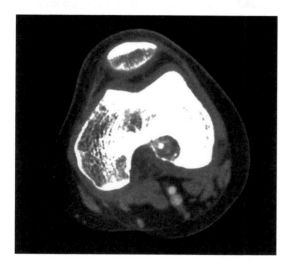

Fig. 28.5 Axial post-contrast CT scan of the left knee in soft tissue window

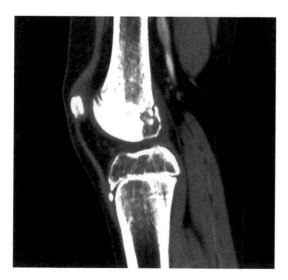

Fig. 28.6 Sagittal post-contrast CT scan of the left knee in soft tissue window

CT images of the left knee demonstrate an oval lytic lesion with internal multiple foci of calcification and no surrounding cortical break. There is a mild heterogeneous enhancement after contrast.

28.3.3 MR Imaging

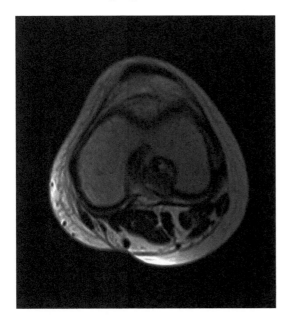

Fig. 28.7 Axial T2 weighted MR image of the left knee

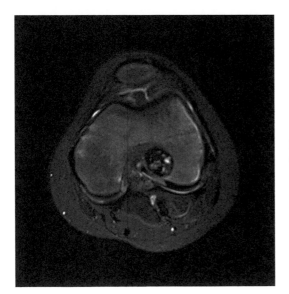

Fig. 28.8 Axial fat-suppressed T2-weighted MR image of the left knee

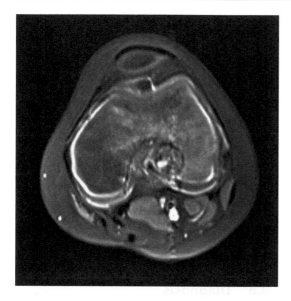

Fig. 28.9 Axial post-contrast fat-suppressed T1-weighted MR image of the left knee

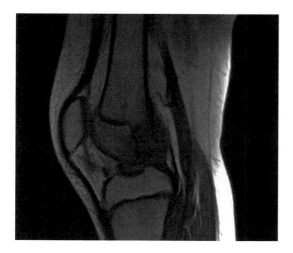

Fig. 28.10 Sagittal T1-weighted MR image of the left knee

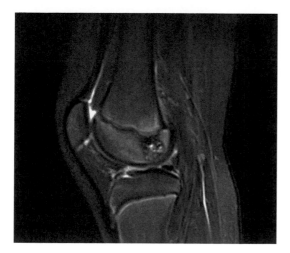

Fig. 28.11 Sagittal fat-suppressed T2-weighted MR image of the left knee

MR images of the left knee demonstrate heterogeneous signal within the lesion. On the T2-weighted images, there are separated areas of lake-like high signal. Heterogeneous mild enhancement is noted on post-contrast images.

28.4 Description and Discussion from Residents

The patient is an adolescent. Radiographs demonstrate small oval area of low density at the distal femoral epiphysis with ill-defined border and no extension across the articular surface. Given the patient's age and imaging findings, chondroblastoma is at the top of the differential diagnosis. Differential diagnosis includes eosinophilic granuloma. On CT scan, the lesion locates at medial aspect of the lateral femoral condyle epiphysis and demonstrates slightly expansile morphology with clear border and thinning of the posterior cortex and internal foci of high densities. Epiphyseal lesion with heterogeneous signal and adjacent marrow edema on MRI and patchy or circular enhancement is noted. The above imaging findings are most indicative of chondroblastoma.

28.5 Analysis and Comments from Professor Cheng Xiao-Guang

This is a typical case in an adolescent with lesion involving the lateral femoral condyle. Chondroblastoma is the most common epiphyseal lesion in adolescent. This case demonstrates typical radiographical, CT and MR findings of chondroblastoma. Lytic lesion with internal multiple foci of calcification with peripheral sclerosis and clear border is noted on radiograph and CT scan. Heterogeneous signal in the lesion on MRI with adjacent marrow edema and mild enhancement are seen. The above imaging findings are pathognomonic of chondroblastoma in a young patient. CT scan can be used to better understand the findings on radiograph. MR images well demonstrate the adjacent marrow edema of reactive changes, characteristic of chondroblastoma.

28.6 Diagnosis

Chondroblastoma.

Suggested Reading

Sailhan F, Chotel F, Parot R. Chondroblastoma of bone in a pediatric population. J Bone Joint Surg Am. 2009;91(9):2159–68.

Weatherall PT, Maale GE, Mendelsohn DB, et al. Chondroblastoma: classic and confusing appearance at MR imaging. Radiology. 1994;190(2):467–74.

Yamamura S, Sato K, Sugiura H, et al. Inflammatory reaction in chondroblastoma. Skelet Radiol. 1996;25(4):371–6.

Chondroblastoma with ABC: Case 4

29.1 Medical History

A 14-year-old boy with right knee pain, restricted activities for a year, and worsening pain with limping for a month.

29.2 Physical Examination

Point tenderness around the right medial femoral condyle.

29.3 Imaging Findings

29.3.1 Radiograph

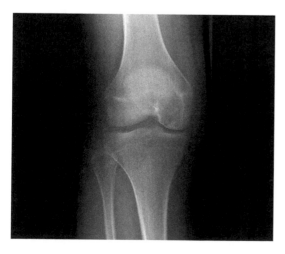

Fig. 29.1 Frontal view of the right knee

© Springer Nature Singapore Pte Ltd. and Peking Union Medical College Press 2020
X. Cheng et al., *Bone Tumor Imaging*, https://doi.org/10.1007/978-981-13-9927-5_29

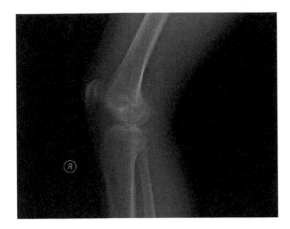

Fig. 29.2 Lateral view of the right knee

Radiographs of the right knee demonstrate low-density lesion in the epiphysis of the right medial femoral condyle with clear border and peripheral sclerosis and internal heterogeneous density.

29.3.2 CT Imaging

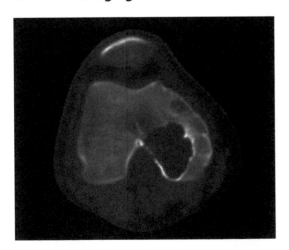

Fig. 29.3 Axial CT scan of the right knee in bone window

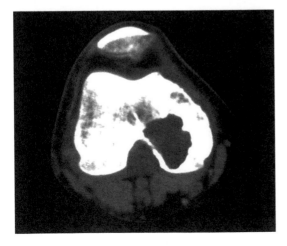

Fig. 29.4 Axial CT scan of the right knee in soft tissue window

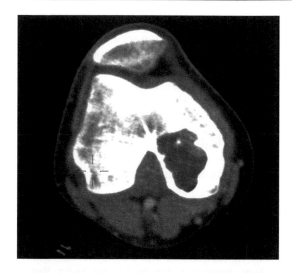

Fig. 29.5 Axial post-contrast CT scan of the right knee in soft tissue window

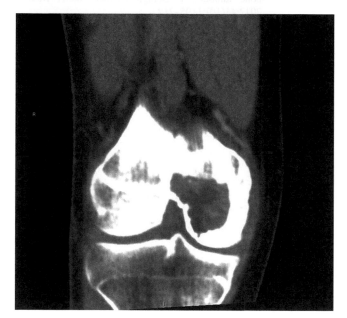

Fig. 29.6 Coronal post-contrast CT scan of the right knee in soft tissue window

CT images of the right knee demonstrate the well-defined and lobulated lytic lesion at the medial femoral condyle with peripheral sclerosis. The lesion appears to be expansile with internal calcification. There is an inhomogeneous enhancement on post-contrast images.

29.4 Description and Discussion from Residents

The patient is an adolescent. Radiographs demonstrate a well-defined lytic lesion in the right medial femoral condyle with peripheral sclerosis.

There is no cortical break or associated soft tissue mass. Given mild soft tissue swelling in the region and patient's age and imaging findings, this is most likely a benign lesion. CT scan demonstrates the lytic lesion with clear sclerotic border, thinning of the cortex without break and internal heterogeneous density with small foci of lobular high densities. There is clear enhancement in the solid area of the lesion, thus likely representing chondroblastoma, with giant cell tumor as differential diagnosis.

29.5 Analysis and Comments from Professor Cheng Xiao-Guang

The patient is an adolescent. The lesion is at the epiphysis of the medial femoral condyle with clear border. Lytic lesion with peripheral sclerosis and internal calcification is noted on CT scan. This is most likely a chondroblastoma with giant cell tumor as differential diagnosis. However, the current lesion is not expansile, and usually there is no internal calcification seen in the lytic lesion of giant cell tumor, thus the current case diagnosis favors chondroblastoma. This is a relatively typical case of chondroblastoma.

29.6 Diagnosis

Chondroblastoma with ABC.

Suggested Reading

Douis H, Saifuddin A. The imaging of cartilaginous bone tumours. I. Benign lesions. Skelet Radiol. 2012;41(10):1195–212.
Sailhan F, Chotel F, Parot R. Chondroblastoma of bone in a pediatric population. J Bone Joint Surg Am. 2009;91(9):2159–68.
Van Dyck P, Vanhoenacker FM, Vogel J, et al. Prevalence, extension and characteristics of fluid-fluid levels in bone and soft tissue tumors. Eur Radiol. 2006;16(12):2644–51.

Myxoid Low-Grade Malignant Mesenchymal Tumor: Case 5

30

30.1 Medical History

A 53-year-old male with dull pain around the right proximal lower leg for 4 years without clear inciting event.

30.2 Physical Examination

Mild swelling around the right knee with an ill-defined hard mass with point tenderness.

30.3 Imaging Findings

30.3.1 Radiograph

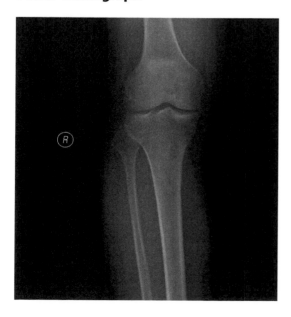

Fig. 30.1 Frontal view of the right knee

© Springer Nature Singapore Pte Ltd. and Peking Union Medical College Press 2020
X. Cheng et al., *Bone Tumor Imaging*, https://doi.org/10.1007/978-981-13-9927-5_30

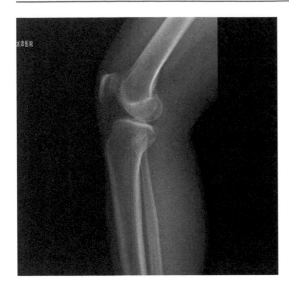

Fig. 30.2 Lateral view of the right knee

Radiographs of the right knee demonstrate a small low-density lesion in the right proximal tibia slightly to the medial aspect. There is a clear border with focal cortical thinning and no periosteal reaction. No clear abnormality is noted in the adjacent soft tissues.

30.3.2 CT Imaging

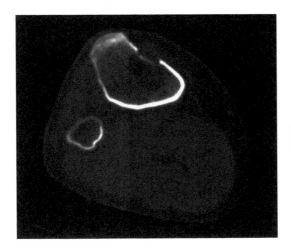

Fig. 30.3 Axial CT scan of the right proximal tibia in bone window

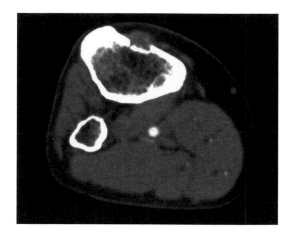

Fig. 30.4 Axial post-contrast CT scan of the right proximal tibia in soft tissue window

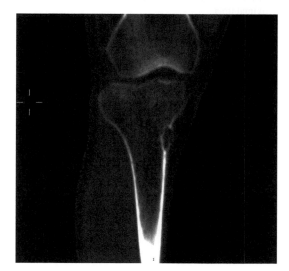

Fig. 30.5 Coronal CT scan of the right proximal tibia in bone window

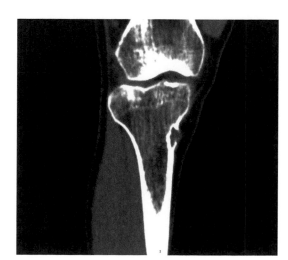

Fig. 30.6 Coronal CT scan of the right proximal tibia in soft tissue window

CT images of the right proximal tibia demonstrate a small, oval, destructive lesion along the medial cortex of the proximal right tibia with internal homogeneous density. There is inhomogeneous enhancement of the soft tissues on post-contrast images.

30.3.3 MR Imaging

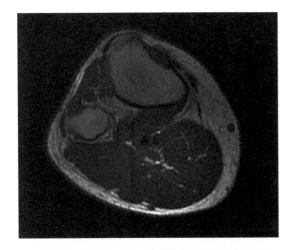

Fig. 30.7 Axial T1-weighted MR image of the right proximal tibia

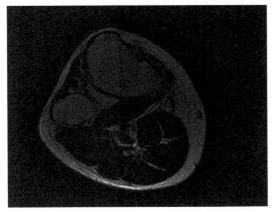

Fig. 30.8 Axial T2-weighted MR image of the right proximal tibia

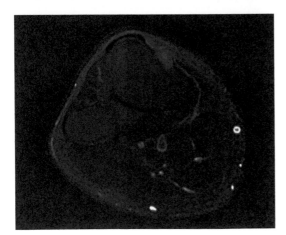

Fig. 30.9 Axial fat-suppressed T2-weighted MR image of the right proximal tibia

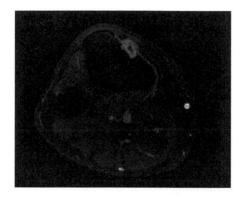

Fig. 30.10 Axial post-contrast fat-suppressed T1-weighted MR image of the right proximal tibia

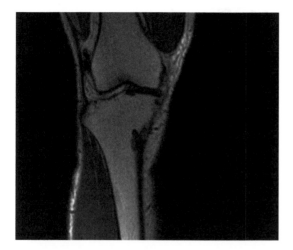

Fig. 30.11 Coronal T1-weighted MR image of the right proximal tibia

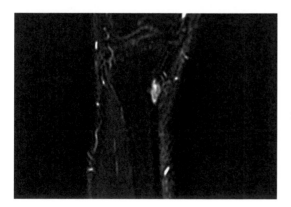

Fig. 30.12 Coronal fat-suppressed T2-weighted MR image of the right proximal tibia

MR images of the right proximal tibia demonstrate isointense T1 and heterogeneous T2 signals of the lytic lesion. On the post-contrast images, there is a heterogeneous enhancement. There is involvement to the medullary cavity.

30.4 Description and Discussion from Residents

The patient is a middle-aged male. Radiographs demonstrate the oval lytic lesion along proximal right tibia with clear border but no peripheral sclerosis and no periosteal reaction or soft tissue mass. Cortical destruction with clear border is demonstrated on CT scan with adjacent cortical thinning and small soft tissue lesion. There is inhomogeneous enhancement. Given the above findings, this is a cortical lesion, likely nonaggressive, of fibrous origin? However, metastatic lesion cannot be excluded. Focal cortical lesion is again demonstrated on MR images. Non enhancing component is also noted in the lesion. Fibrous lesion is in the differential diagnosis; metastatic lesion cannot be excluded.

30.5 Analysis and Comments from Professor Cheng Xiao-Guang

Focal cortical lesion without internal calcification but with inhomogeneous densities in a middle-aged male with prolonged clinical course; tumor with myxoid component cannot be excluded. Some radiologists consider fibrous lesion; however, fibrous lesion is rare after closure of the physis. The patient presented with pain in the region, and there appears to be abundant blood supply to the lesion, raising concern for aggressive lesion. Overall, the lesion demonstrates nonspecific imaging findings with differential diagnosis including benign lesion such as Langerhans cell histiocytosis and malignant lesion. Biopsy with tissue sampling is recommended.

30.6 Diagnosis

Myxoid low-grade malignant mesenchymal tumor.

Suggested Reading

Levine SM, Lambiase RE, Petchprapa CN. Cortical lesions of the tibia: characteristic appearances at conventional radiography. Radiographics. 2003;23(1):157–77.
Sade R, Yuce I, Karaca L, et al. Malignant mesenchymal tumor of the sacrum. Spine J. 2015;15(10): e39–40.

31.1 Medical History

A 15-year-old boy with history of injury.

31.2 Physical Examination

No abnormality.

31.3 Imaging Findings

31.3.1 Radiograph

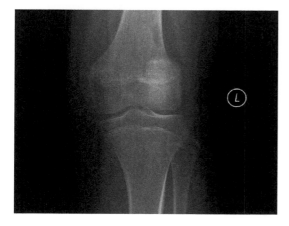

Fig. 31.1 Frontal view of the left knee

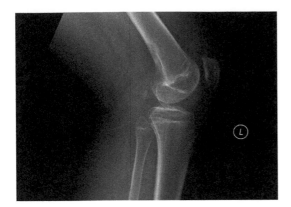

Fig. 31.2 Lateral view of the left knee

Radiographs of the left knee demonstrate cortical buckling along the left distal femur posteriorly.

31.3.2 CT Imaging

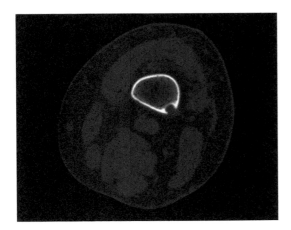

Fig. 31.3 Axial CT scan of the left knee in bone window

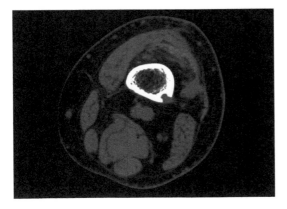

Fig. 31.4 Axial CT scan of the left knee in soft tissue window

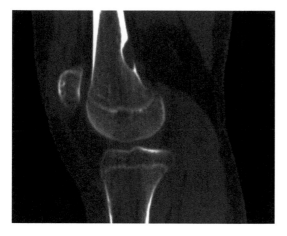

Fig. 31.5 Sagittal CT scan of the left knee in bone window

CT images of the left knee demonstrate focal lytic lesion along the posterior distal femoral cortex with peripheral sclerosis.

31.4 Description and Discussion from Residents

The patient is an adolescent. Radiographs demonstrate a well-defined lesion along the cortex of the posterior distal femur with mild sclerosis and thinning of the cortex. On CT scan, the lesion just involves the cortex with homogeneous density and mild peripheral sclerosis and no clear soft tissue mass. Given the above imaging findings and the patient's age and region of involvement, this is a typical case of fibrous cortical defect.

31.5 Analysis and Comments from Professor Cheng Xiao-Guang

Focal well-defined cortical lesion with homogeneous density in an adolescent patient is a typical presentation of focal fibrous cortical defect. However, this needs to be differentiated from nonossifying fibroma and cortical desmoid. Nonossifying fibroma and focal fibrous cortical defect are same entity pathologically; the only differences are on imaging. Larger lesion with big diameter (>3 cm) which involves the medullary cavity is classified as non-ossifying fibroma. Smaller lesion that just involves the cortex is called fibrous cortical defect. It is important to emphasis that fibrous cortical defect is a self-limiting process without need for treatment. Cortical desmoid is likely related to injury or growth and commonly affects myotendinous attachment at posterior medial aspect of distal femur. It usually demonstrates as a lesion protrudes from outside to the cortex. Some believe that cortical desmoid is a manifestation of fibrous cortical defect when there is less cellular component.

31.6 Diagnosis

Fibrous cortical defect.

Suggested Reading

Betsy M, Kupersmith LM, Springfield DS. Metaphyseal fibrous defects. J Am Acad Orthop Surg. 2004;12(2):89–95.
Ritschl P, Karnel F, Hajek P. Fibrous metaphyseal defects—determination of their origin and natural history using a radiomorphological study. Skelet Radiol. 1988;17(1):8–15.

Fibrous Cortical Defect: Case 7

32

32.1 Medical History

A 16-year-old boy with no complains.

32.2 Physical Examination

No abnormality.

32.3 Imaging Findings

32.3.1 CT Imaging

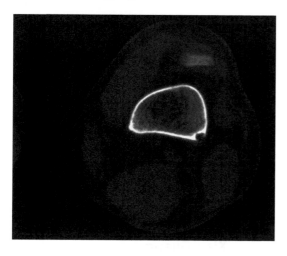

Fig. 32.1 Axial CT scan of the left knee in bone window

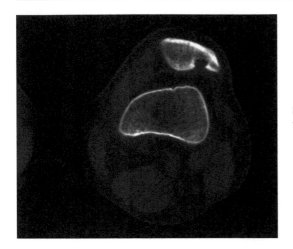

Fig. 32.2 Axial CT scan of the left knee in bone window

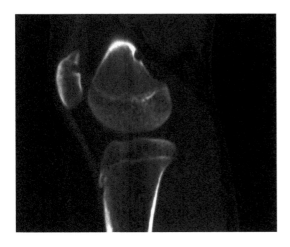

Fig. 32.3 Sagittal CT scan of the left knee in bone window

CT images of the left knee demonstrate focal cortical defect along the posterior metaphysis of the left distal femur and the lateral aspect of the patella.

32.4 Description and Discussion from Residents

The patient is an adolescent boy. There are focal lesions along the articular surface of the patella and posterior distal femur. The two lesions are well-defined with homogeneous density and without soft tissue mass. Based on imaging findings, these are benign lesions: The lesion at the femur is fibrous cortical defect and the lesion at the patella is dorsal defect of the patella. However, some residents thought these lesions could be of same etiology.

32.5 Analysis and Comments from Professor Cheng Xiao-Guang

Focal well-defined lesions with internal homogeneous density and involvements of multiple bones in an adolescent patient most likely are a benign process. Usually when there are multiple bone involvements with similar imaging characteristics, they are of same etiology. However, the femoral lesion of the current case is very typical for fibrous cortical defect. Though, fibrous cortical defect is very rare in patella. Dorsal defect of the patella is favored to the diagnosis of this patella lesion. Dorsal defect of the patella is of unknown etiology and likely a normal developmental anomaly of the patella. The lesion usually manifests as cortical defect along dorsal patella with intact overlying cartilage.

32.6 Diagnosis

Fibrous cortical defect of distal femur, dorsal defect of the patella.

Suggested Reading

Ritschl P, Karnel F, Hajek P. Fibrous metaphyseal defects—determination of their origin and natural history using a radiomorphological study. Skelet Radiol. 1988;17(1):8–15.

van Holsbeeck M, Vandamme B, Marchal G, et al. Dorsal defect of the patella: concept of its origin and relationship with bipartite and multipartite patella. Skelet Radiol. 1987;16(4):304–11.

33.1 Medical History

A 32-year-old female with left distal femoral lesion seen on radiograph of the left knee for patella fracture 4 years ago and no clinical complaint.

33.2 Physical Examination

No abnormality.

33.3 Imaging Findings

33.3.1 MR Imaging

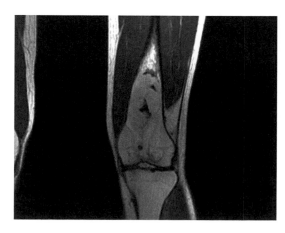

Fig. 33.1 Coronal T1-weighted MR image of the left distal femur

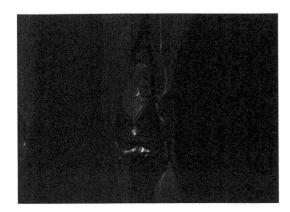

Fig. 33.2 Coronal fat-suppressed T2-weighted MR image of the left distal femur

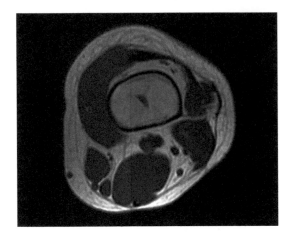

Fig. 33.3 Axial T1-weighted MR image of the left distal femur

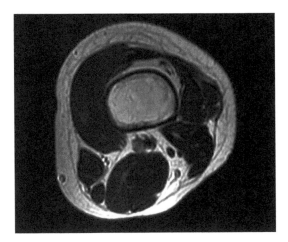

Fig. 33.4 Axial T2-weighted MR image of the left distal femur

MR images of the left distal femur demonstrate a lesion within the distal femoral intramedullary canal and mildly expansile. It measured about 10.5 cm × 4.3 cm × 3.0 cm. The inferior margin of the lesion is close to the articular surface. The lesion demonstrates T1 and T2 high signal and low signal on fat-suppressed T2-weighted images. There are multiple foci of irregular low signal within the lesion and surrounded by high signal on fat-suppressed T2-weighted images. There is thinning of the adjacent cortex without break. No abnormal signal is noted in the adjacent musculatures.

33.4 Description and Discussion from Residents

The patient is a young female with relatively long clinical course. There is a mildly expansile lesion at the distal femur with intact cortex and clear border on MR images. No soft tissue mass, periosteal reaction, or marrow edema is noted. Based on the above imaging findings, this is most likely a benign process. Majority of the lesion demonstrates high T1 and T2 signals with low signal on fat-suppressed sequences, consistent with fatty tissue. There is internal linear long T1 and long T2 signal, likely of cystic changes. Given majority of the lesion demonstrates fat signal, this is intra-osseous lipoma.

33.5 Analysis and Comments from Professor Cheng Xiao-Guang

A mildly expansile lesion at the distal femur with heterogeneous signal but majority of fat signal and in a young female patient is most consistent with intra-osseous lipoma. But we need to emphasize here that for bone and joint lesions, especially of bone tumor cases, the diagnosis needs to be based on radiograph, CT scan, and MR images together. Radiograph and CT scan are critical at evaluating bone and joint disease, with clear advantage at delineating cortical destruction and presence of calcification within the lesion. Majority of bone tumors demonstrate nonspecific findings on MR images, and diagnosis needs to be made with correlation with radiograph or CT scan.

33.6 Diagnosis

Intra-osseous lipoma.

Suggested Reading

Campbell RS, Grainger AJ, Mangham DC, et al. Intraosseous lipoma: report of 35 new cases and a review of the literature. Skelet Radiol. 2003;32(4):209–22.
Milgram JW. Malignant transformation in bone lipomas. Skelet Radiol. 1990;19(5):347–52.

34

34.1 Medical History

A 17-year-old girl with left lower leg pain for 1½ month and worsen with palpable mass for half a month.

34.2 Physical Examination

Mild swelling around left proximal fibula with focal palpable, hard mass, and point tenderness.

34.3 Imaging Findings

34.3.1 MR Imaging

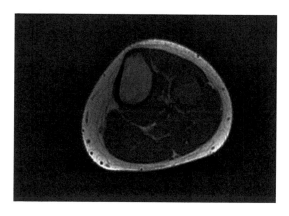

Fig. 34.1 Axial T1-weighted MR image of the left proximal fibula

© Springer Nature Singapore Pte Ltd. and Peking Union Medical College Press 2020
X. Cheng et al., *Bone Tumor Imaging*, https://doi.org/10.1007/978-981-13-9927-5_34

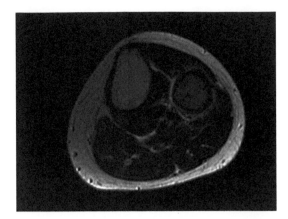

Fig. 34.2 Axial T2-weighted MR image of the left proximal fibula

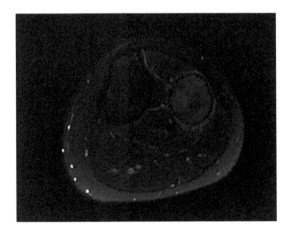

Fig. 34.3 Axial fat-suppressed T2-weighted MR image of the left proximal fibula

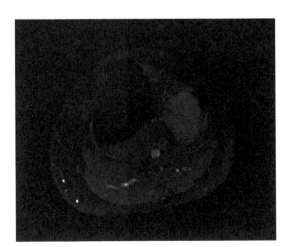

Fig. 34.4 Axial post-contrast fat-suppressed T1-weighted MR image of the left proximal fibula

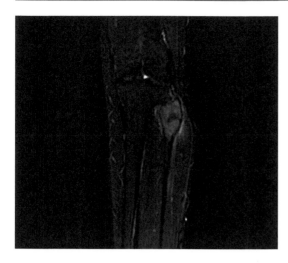

Fig. 34.5 Coronal fat-suppressed T2-weighted MR image of left proximal fibula

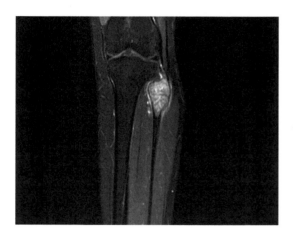

Fig. 34.6 Coronal post-contrast fat-suppressed T1-weighted MR image of the left proximal fibula

MR images of the left proximal fibula demonstrate an expansile destructive lesion. There are internal low T1, mildly high T2 signals and heterogeneous high signal on fat-suppressed sequence with avid enhancement. Mild surrounding soft tissue edema is noted.

avid enhancement. End of bone lesion with expansile destruction and avid enhancement is consistent with giant cell tumor. However, the patient is relatively young, differential diagnosis include PNET (primitive neuroectodermal tumor).

34.4   Description and Discussion from Residents

The patient is an adolescent girl with expansile destructive lesion at the fibular head. The lesion is well-defined without soft tissue swelling and demonstrates low T1 and high T2 signals with

34.5   Analysis and Comments from Professor Cheng Xiao-Guang

Expansile bony destructive lesion at fibular head with avid enhancement and in a young female patient is consistent with giant cell tumor of bone. However, we need to emphasize that for bone and joint disease, especially bone tumor cases, usually with nonspecific findings on MRI, the diagnosis needs to be made combining the findings from radiograph and CT scan.

34.6   Diagnosis

Giant cell tumor of bone.

Suggested Reading

Chakarun CJ, Forrester DM, Gottsegen CJ, et al. Giant cell tumor of bone: review, mimics, and new developments in treatment. Radiographics. 2013;33(1):197–211.

Denison GL, Workman TL. General case of the day. Benign giant cell tumor with extension through the fibular head into the adjacent soft tissue. Radiographics. 1997;17(2):545–7.

Murphey MD, Nomikos GC, Flemming DJ, et al. From the archives of AFIP. Imaging of giant cell tumor and giant cell reparative granuloma of bone: radiologic-pathologic correlation. Radiographics. 2001;21(5):1283–309.

Osteosarcoma: Case 10

35.1 Medical History

A 59-year-old male with pain and swelling at distal right thigh for more than a month.

35.2 Physical Examination

Mild swelling around right distal thigh with focal point tenderness.

35.3 Imaging Findings

35.3.1 Radiograph

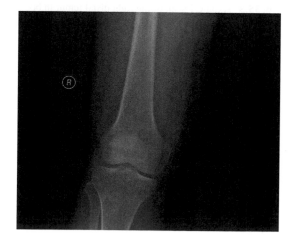

Fig. 35.1 Frontal view of the right knee

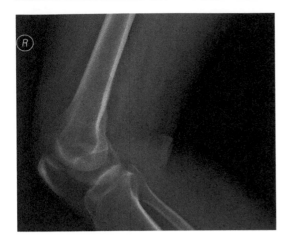

Fig. 35.2 Lateral view of the right knee

Radiographs of the right knee demonstrate lytic bony destruction at right distal femur with clear border and no periosteal reaction.

35.3.2 CT Imaging

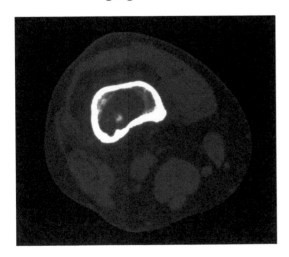

Fig. 35.3 Axial CT scan of the right distal femur in bone window

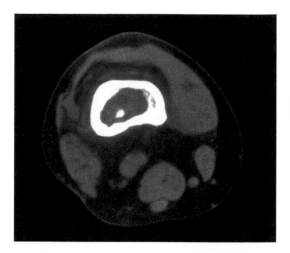

Fig. 35.4 Axial CT scan of the right distal femur in soft tissue window

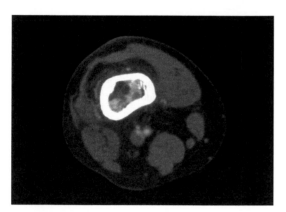

Fig. 35.5 Axial post-contrast CT scan of the right distal femur in soft tissue window

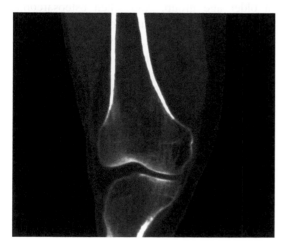

Fig. 35.6 Coronal CT scan of the right distal femur in bone window

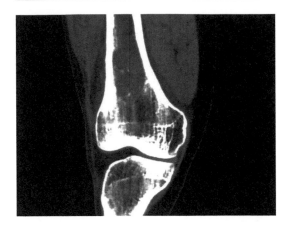

Fig. 35.7 Coronal CT scan of the right distal femur in soft tissue window

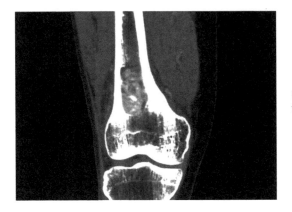

Fig. 35.8 Coronal post-contrast CT scan of the right distal femur in soft tissue window

CT images of the right distal femur demonstrate lytic process of the medullary cavity with internal scattered high densities. There is soft tissue mass extending outside of the cortex. The border is not clear. On the post-contrast images, there is avid enhancement in the solid area with area of necrosis noted.

35.4   Description and Discussion from Residents

The patient is a middle-aged man. Radiographs demonstrate lytic lesion of the right distal femur with cortical destruction. The lesion is noted to involve the medullary cavity on CT scan with internal multiple calcifications. There are also cortical thinning and avid enhancement. The above findings are not consistent of typical chondrosarcoma imaging findings. Osteosarcoma is

commonly seen in adolescents but can be seen in older age group. And when osteosarcoma occurs in older age group, the imaging findings are usually not typical. Thus, besides including metastatic lesion in the differential diagnosis, osteosarcoma should also be included. Additionally, undifferentiated high-grade pleomorphic sarcoma or dedifferentiated chondrosarcoma should also be included in the differential diagnosis.

35.5   Analysis and Comments from Professor Cheng Xiao-Guang

The patient is a 59-year-old male with lesion at right distal femoral diaphysis without clear border on radiograph. Cortical destruction with ill-defined border and internal multiple high densities is noted on CT scan. This could be considered as chondrosarcoma based on radiograph and non-contrast CT scan images. However, there is avid enhancement focally with CT value of 170–180HU, not supportive of the diagnosis of chondrosarcoma. Additionally, there is an adjacent soft tissue edema with thickened vessels and ill-defined margin. Overall, this is a malignant lesion. Given the patient's age, undifferentiated high-grade pleomorphic sarcoma is first considered, and osteosarcoma is included in the differential diagnosis.

35.6 Diagnosis

Osteosarcoma (rare type: osteoblastoma-like osteosarcoma).

Suggested Reading

Abramovici L, Kenan S, Hytiroglou P, et al. Osteoblastoma-like osteosarcoma of the distal tibia. Skelet Radiol. 2002;31(3):179–82.

Gambarotti M, Dei Tos AP, Vanel D, et al. Osteoblastoma-like osteosarcoma: high-grade or low-grade osteosarcoma? Histopathology. 2019;74(3):494–503.

36.1 Medical History

A 46-year-old male with right knee transient weakness for more than 70 days.

36.2 Physical Examination

Mild swelling around the right knee.

36.3 Imaging Findings

36.3.1 Radiograph

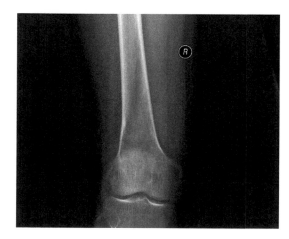

Fig. 36.1 Frontal view of the right distal femur

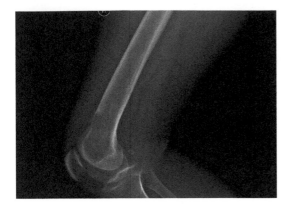

Fig. 36.2 Lateral view of the right distal femur

Radiographs of the right distal femur demonstrate anterior lytic lesion at the metaphysis of the distal femur with cortical break and without sclerotic border.

36.3.2 CT Imaging

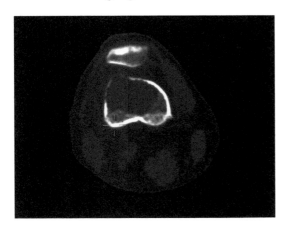

Fig. 36.3 Axial CT scan of the right knee in bone window

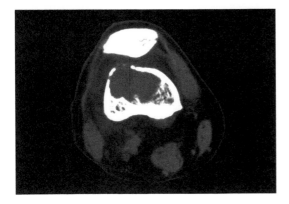

Fig. 36.4 Axial CT scan of the right knee in soft tissue window

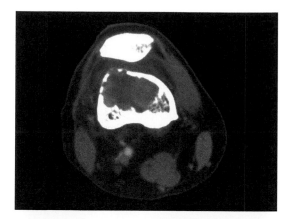

Fig. 36.5 Axial post-contrast CT image of the right knee in soft tissue window

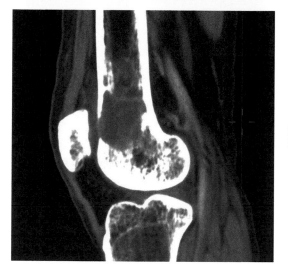

Fig. 36.6 Sagittal post-contrast CT image of the right knee in soft tissue window

CT images of the right knee demonstrate lytic lesion at the distal femur without clear margin and no clear periosteal reaction. The internal CT value of the lesion is about 42HU. There is inhomogeneous enhancement.

36.3.3 MR Imaging

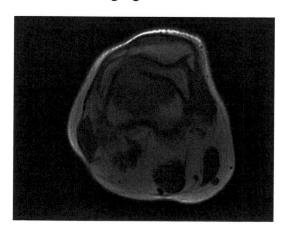

Fig. 36.7 Axial T1-weighted MR image of the right knee

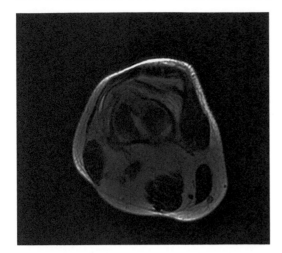

Fig. 36.8 Axial T2-weighted MR image of the right knee

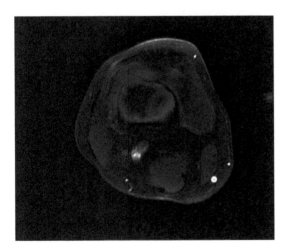

Fig. 36.9 Axial post-contrast fat-suppressed T1-weighted MR image of right knee

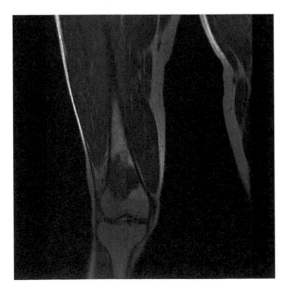

Fig. 36.10 Coronal T1-weighted MR image of the right knee

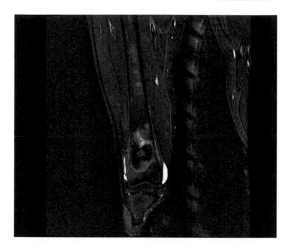

Fig. 36.11 Coronal fat-suppressed T2-weighted MR image of the right knee

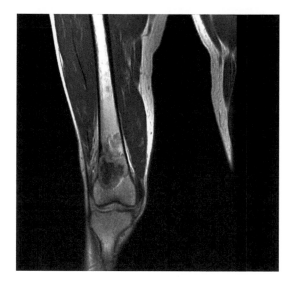

Fig. 36.12 Coronal post-contrast T1-weighted MR image of the left knee

MR images of the right knee demonstrate the lesion in the right distal femur. There is an associated soft tissue mass extending from the cortical break with internal heterogeneous signal. At the center of the lesion, there are low T1 and T2 signals, and within the peripheral of the lesion, there are slightly low T1 and high T2 signals. Heterogeneous enhancement is noted with surrounding marrow edema.

36.4 Description and Discussion from Residents

The patient is a middle-aged male. Radiographs demonstrate lytic lesion of the right distal femur with cortical break and unclear margin. There is

an irregular cortex anteriorly of mild periosteal reaction and surrounding soft tissue swelling. On CT scan, there is internal punctate calcification within the lesion. There is an ill-defined margin of the lesion with periosteal reaction. Soft tissue mass is noted to extend through anterior cortical break. Mild heterogeneous enhancement is noted. Internal low T1 signal is noted on MR images of the lesion with linear low signal seen on fat-suppressed sequences. Heterogeneous signals are noted on T2-weighted sequences, mostly of iso and low signals. Peripheral avid enhancement is noted. Given the above constellation of findings, undifferentiated high-grade pleomorphic sarcoma is the likely diagnosis and osteosarcoma, small round cell tumors are in the differential diagnosis.

36.5 Analysis and Comments from Professor Cheng Xiao-Guang

Bony destructive lesion at the right distal femoral metaphysis with ill-defined border is noted. On the lateral view radiograph, there is ill-defined margin at the supra-patellar region, of cortical break. Calcification inside of the lesion is noted on CT scan with mild heterogeneous enhancement. CT value of the avid enhancement area is 80HU. MR images demonstrate the extent of the lesion in more detail. This is a malignant lesion, with differential diagnosis including undifferentiated high-grade pleomorphic sarcoma, osteosarcoma, and metastatic lesion.

36.6 Diagnosis

Undifferentiated high-grade pleomorphic sarcoma (malignant fibrous histiocytoma of bone).

Suggested Reading

Koplas MC, Lefkowitz RA, Bauer TW. Imaging findings, prevalence and outcome of de novo and secondary malignant fibrous histiocytoma of bone. Skelet Radiol. 2010;39(8):791–8.

Link TM, Haeussler MD, Poppek S, et al. Malignant fibrous histiocytoma of bone: conventional X-ray and MR imaging features. Skelet Radiol. 1998;27(10):552–8.

37.1 Medical History

A 31-year-old male with persistent pain of the left knee without clear inciting event for 2 months and worsening for 1 month.

37.2 Physical Examination

Left lower leg swelling with redness and warmth of the anterior skin of proximal left lower leg. No palpable mass noted.

37.3 Imaging Findings

37.3.1 Radiograph

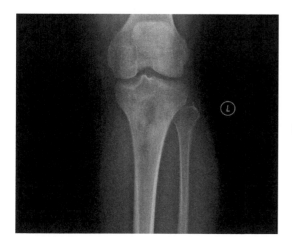

Fig. 37.1 Frontal view of the left knee

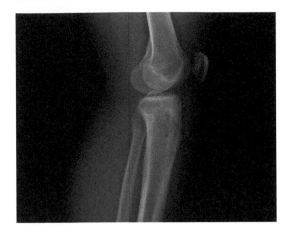

Fig. 37.2 Lateral view of the left knee

Radiographs of the left knee demonstrate bone destruction along the proximal left tibia without clear margin. Periosteal reaction and adjacent soft tissue swelling are noted.

37.3.2 CT Imaging

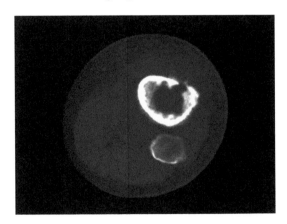

Fig. 37.3 Axial CT scan of the left knee in bone window

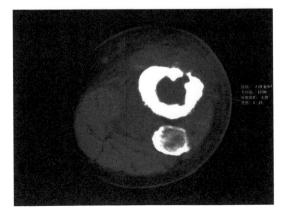

Fig. 37.4 Axial CT scan of the left knee in soft tissue window

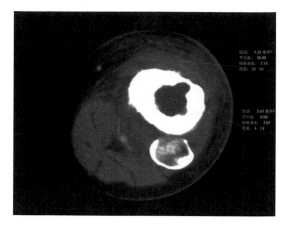

Fig. 37.5 Axial post-contrast CT image of the left knee in soft tissue window

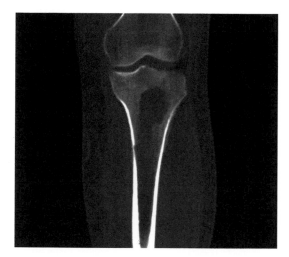

Fig. 37.6 Coronal CT image of the left knee in bone window

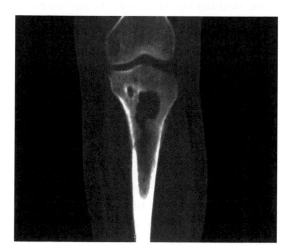

Fig. 37.7 Coronal CT image of the left knee in bone window

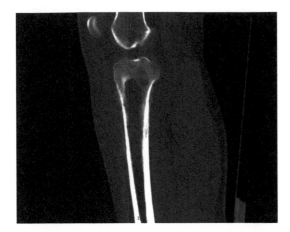

Fig. 37.8 Sagittal CT image of the left knee in bone window

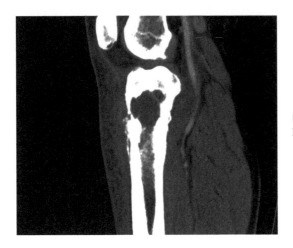

Fig. 37.9 Sagittal post-contrast CT image of the left knee in soft tissue window

CT images of the left knee demonstrate bony destruction around the proximal left tibial metaphysis with surrounding sclerosis and extensive periosteal reaction. There is low CT value internally and no clear enhancement. Adjacent soft tissue swelling is noted.

37.4 Description and Discussion from Residents

The patient is a young male. Left proximal tibial bone destruction with periosteal reaction and adjacent soft tissue swelling with strands of the subcutaneous soft tissue are noted on the radiograph and most suggestive of infectious etiology. Left proximal tibial bone destruction with sclerosis and focal smooth periosteal reaction and soft

tissue swelling and strands of the subcutaneous soft tissue are noted on CT scan. There is suggestion of sinus track and enhancement in the solid portion of the lesion. The above findings are most consistent with osteomyelitis.

37.5 Analysis and Comments from Professor Cheng Xiao-Guang

The patient is a young male. Radiographs demonstrate left proximal tibial bone destruction with periosteal reaction and adjacent soft tissue swelling, most suggestive of infectious etiology. Multiple areas of bone destruction at left proximal tibia with periosteal reaction and soft tissue swelling and focal peripheral enhancement with more area of central no enhancement are seen on CT scan. Osteomyelitis is first in the differential diagnosis with rather typical imaging findings; however, osteosarcoma cannot be entirely excluded.

37.6 Diagnosis

Osteomyelitis.

Suggested Reading

Beaman FD, von Herrmann PF, Kransdorf MJ, et al. ACR appropriateness criteria® suspected osteomyelitis, septic arthritis, or soft tissue infection (excluding spine and diabetic foot). J Am Coll Radiol. 2017;14(5S):S326–37.

Lee YJ, Sadigh S, Mankad K, et al. The imaging of osteomyelitis. Quant Imaging Med Surg. 2016;6(2):184–98.

Synovial Sarcoma: Case 13

38.1 Medical History

A 24-year-old female with pain and discomfort around the left lower leg for 5 months and palpable mass recently.

38.2 Physical Examination

Palpable mass along the medial aspect of the left lower leg, hard, without clear border, and non-movable.

38.3 Imaging Findings

38.3.1 Radiograph

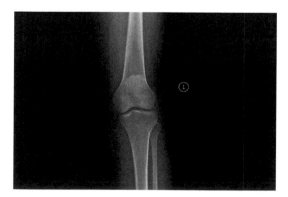

Fig. 38.1 Frontal view of the left knee

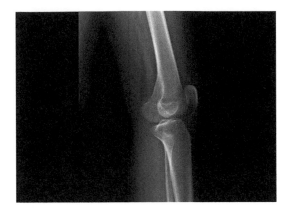

Fig. 38.2 Lateral view of the left knee

Radiographs of the left knee demonstrate a soft tissue mass along the medial aspect of the left proximal tibia.

38.3.2 MR Imaging

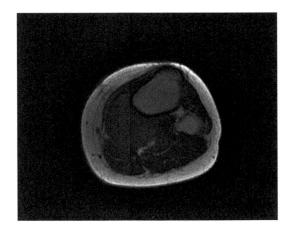

Fig. 38.3 Axial T1-weighted MR image of the left knee

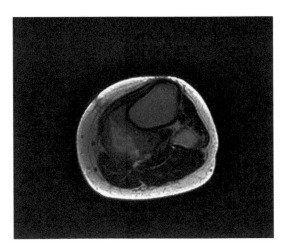

Fig. 38.4 Axial T2-weighted MR image of the left knee

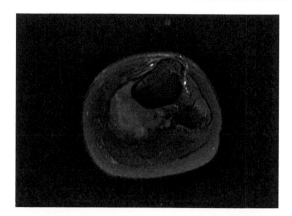

Fig. 38.5 Axial fat-suppressed T2-weighted MR image of the left knee

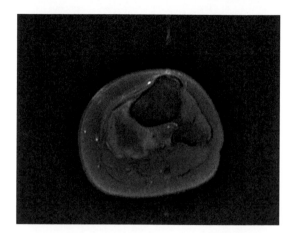

Fig. 38.6 Axial post-contrast fat-suppressed T1-weighted MR image of the left knee

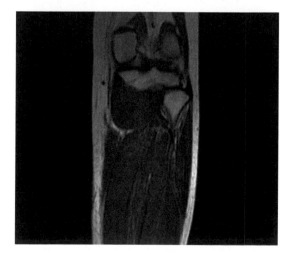

Fig. 38.7 Coronal T1-weighted MR image of the left knee

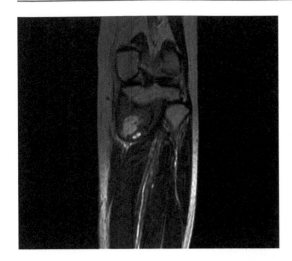

Fig. 38.8 Coronal T2-weighted MR image of the left knee

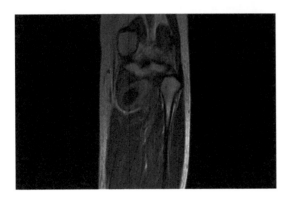

Fig. 38.9 Coronal post-contrast T1-weighted MR image of the left knee

MR images of the left knee demonstrate the soft tissue mass around the medial and posterior aspect of the left proximal tibia. The lesion demonstrates low T1 and heterogeneous high T2 signals. There are internal necrosis and cystic changes with peripheral enhancement.

38.4   Description and Discussion from Residents

The patient is a young female. Radiographs demonstrate soft tissue density abutting the medial aspect of the left proximal tibia with clear margin from the underlying cortex. The lesion demonstrates low signal on T1-weighted sequences and internal central high T2 signal with peripheral low signal on T2-weighted sequences. Peripheral enhancement is noted on the post-contrast images. Given the above findings, this is most likely a soft tissue tumor, and adjacent to the joint, synovial sarcoma is a possibility. Organizing hematoma and myositis ossificans are in the differential diagnoses.

38.5   Analysis and Comments from Professor Cheng Xiao-Guang

The soft tissue mass demonstrates rather homogenous density on radiograph. On the MRI images, the lesion is abutting the tibial cortex and surrounds it in medial and posterior aspect. There is no invasion of the cortex or periosteal reaction. If this is a soft tissue tumor, it is most likely synovial sarcoma. Since there is a sharp angle of the lesion with adjacent cortex, we also need to include bone surface tumor and tumor from the periosteum in the differential diagnosis, such as periosteal osteosarcoma. Since there is no circumferential calcification proceeding from outer margins toward the center noted on radiograph or CT of "egg shell like calcification," myositis ossificans can be excluded.

38.6 Diagnosis

Synovial sarcoma.

Suggested Reading

Bakri A, Shinagare AB, Krajewski KM, et al. Synovial sarcoma: imaging features of common and uncommon primary sites, metastatic patterns, and treatment response. AJR Am J Roentgenol. 2012;199(2):W208–15.

Murphey MD, Gibson MS, Jennings BT, et al. From the archives of the AFIP: imaging of synovial sarcoma with radiologic-pathologic correlation. Radiographics. 2006;26(5):1543–65.

Synovial Sarcoma: Case 14

39.1 Medical History

A 16-year-old boy with right knee swelling and pain for 3 years.

39.2 Physical Examination

Palpable mass along the lateral aspect of right distal femur.

39.3 Imaging Findings

39.3.1 Radiograph

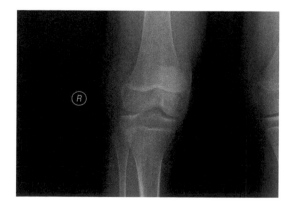

Fig. 39.1 Frontal view of the right knee

© Springer Nature Singapore Pte Ltd. and Peking Union Medical College Press 2020
X. Cheng et al., *Bone Tumor Imaging*, https://doi.org/10.1007/978-981-13-9927-5_39

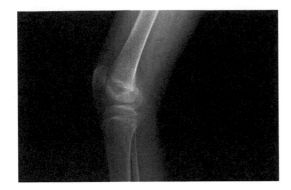

Fig. 39.2 Lateral view of the right knee

Radiographs of the right knee demonstrate soft tissue swelling along the distal right femur laterally.

39.3.2 CT Imaging

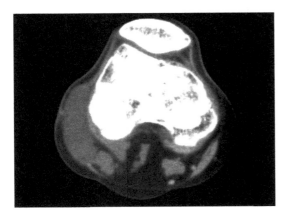

Fig. 39.3 Axial CT image of the right knee in soft tissue window

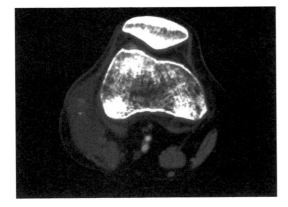

Fig. 39.4 Axial post-contrast CT image of the right knee in soft tissue window

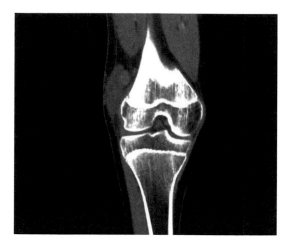

Fig. 39.5 Coronal post-contrast CT image of the right knee in soft tissue window

CT images of the right knee demonstrate mass-like soft tissue lesion along the distal femur laterally with homogenous density and no clear margin. Focal enhancement is noted after contrast injection.

39.3.3 MR Imaging

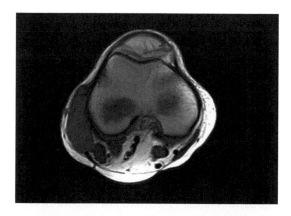

Fig. 39.6 Axial T1-weighted MR image of the right knee

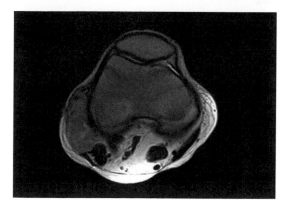

Fig. 39.7 Axial T2-weighted MR image of the right knee

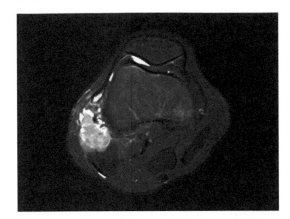

Fig. 39.8 Axial fat-suppressed T2-weighted MR image of the right knee

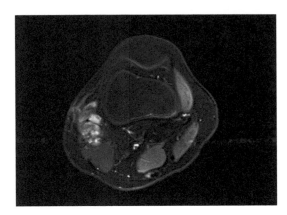

Fig. 39.9 Axial post-contrast fat-suppressed T1-weighted MR image of the right knee

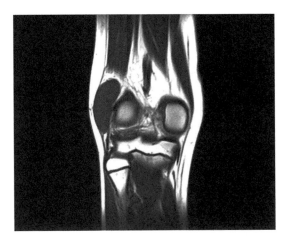

Fig. 39.10 Coronal T1-weighted MR image of the right knee

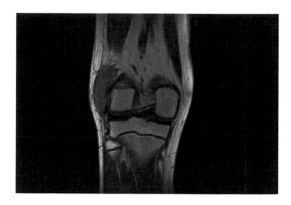

Fig. 39.11 Coronal post-contrast T1-weighted MR image of the right knee

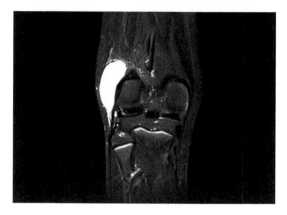

Fig. 39.12 Coronal fat-suppressed T2-weighted MR image of the right knee

MR images of the right knee demonstrate the soft tissue mass at lateral aspect of the right knee with isointense T1 signal and high T2 signal with enhancement.

39.4 Description and Discussion from Residents

The patient is an adolescent. Radiographs demonstrate soft tissue density abutting the lateral distal right femur. On the CT scan, there is punctate calcification within the soft tissue mass with irregular margin from underlying subcutaneous soft tissue and mild periosteal reaction along lateral distal femur. Enhancement is also seen. On MR images, there are heterogeneous T2 signal within the lesion and internal septations and nodular low signals. There is a suggestion of close relationship of the soft tissue lesion with the knee joint capsule. The above imaging findings are suggestive of synovial sarcoma; giant cell tumor of the tendon sheath and hemangioma are in the differential diagnosis.

39.5 Analysis and Comments from Professor Cheng Xiao-Guang

Soft tissue mass along the right knee laterally with lobular contour and internal calcification with close relationship to the joint capsule without clear invasion, hemangioma is at the top of the differential diagnosis. However, hemangioma usually is not well circumscribed with phlebolith on radiograph and linear flow voids noted on MRI, not seen in the current case. Differential diagnosis is synovial sarcoma, which is usually outside the joint but adjacent and hard to distinguish from other soft tissue tumors, and not highly invasive.

39.6 Diagnosis

Synovial sarcoma.

Suggested Reading

Bakri A, Shinagare AB, Krajewski KM, et al. Synovial sarcoma: imaging features of common and uncommon primary sites, metastatic patterns, and treatment response. AJR Am J Roentgenol. 2012;199(2):W208–15.

Murphey MD, Gibson MS, Jennings BT, et al. From the archives of the AFIP: imaging of synovial sarcoma with radiologic-pathologic correlation. Radiographics. 2006;26(5):1543–65.

Pigmented Villonodular Synovitis (PVNS): Case 15

40

40.1 Medical History

A 28-year-old female with left knee palpable mass for 2 years and worsening with pain and limited activities for 3 months.

40.2 Physical Examination

Swelling around the left knee without clear margin and mild point tenderness.

40.3 Imaging Findings

40.3.1 Radiograph

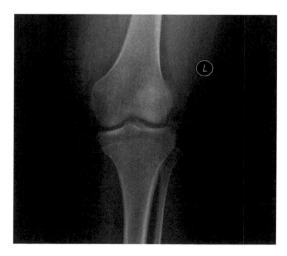

Fig. 40.1 Frontal view of the left knee

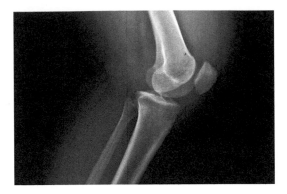

Fig. 40.2 Lateral view of the left knee

Radiographs of the left knee demonstrate soft tissue swelling and prominence at the supra-patellar region.

40.3.2 MR Imaging

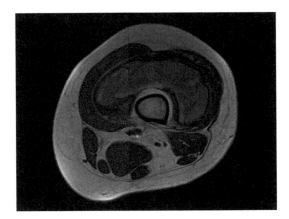

Fig. 40.3 Axial T1-weighted MR image of the left knee

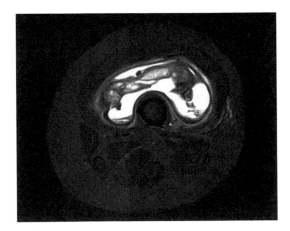

Fig. 40.4 Axial fat-suppressed T2-weighted MR image of the left knee

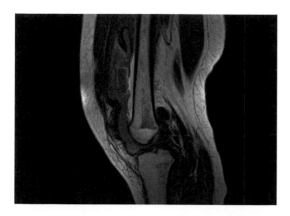

Fig. 40.5 Sagittal T1-weighted MR image of the left knee

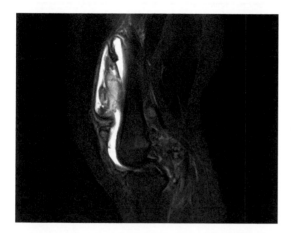

Fig. 40.6 Sagittal fat-suppressed T2-weighted MR image of the left knee

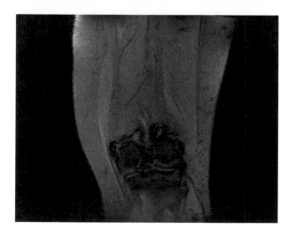

Fig. 40.7 Coronal gradient echo MR image of the left knee

MR images of the left knee demonstrate large left knee effusion with synovial hyperplasia and internal linear low signal on all sequences with blooming on gradient echo sequence. Soft tissue edema is also present.

40.4   Description and Discussion from Residents

The patient is a young female. Radiographs demonstrate soft tissue prominence around the left knee without cortical destruction. There are increased soft tissue densities in supra-patellar, infra-patellar, and popliteal regions. The articular surface of the left knee is preserved. Extensive synovial hyperplasia with large effusion is noted on MR images. High T1 signal is noted, indicating hemorrhage. Linear low signals on all sequences could represent hemosiderin, especially with blooming on gradient echo sequences. The above findings are most suggestive of pigmented villonodular synovitis (PVNS); differential diagnosis includes hemophilia.

40.5   Analysis and Comments from Professor Cheng Xiao-Guang

Radiographs demonstrate normal osseous structures of the knee with soft tissue prominence and loss of normal lucent fatty tissue at the infra-patellar region and indistinct quadriceps tendon. Synovial hyperplasia with large effusion is seen on MR images with local high T1 signal of hemorrhage and linear low signals on all sequences, with blooming on gradient echo sequences, indicating hemosiderin. Given the above imaging findings and patient's history, the top diagnosis is PVNS, with typical imaging findings. Differential diagnosis is hemangioma, usually with internal flow voids, not seen in the current case.

40.6   Diagnosis

Pigmented villonodular synovitis (tenosynovial giant cell tumor, diffuse type).

Suggested Reading

Cheng XG, You YH, Liu W, et al. MRI features of pigmented villonodular synovitis (PVNS). Clin Rheumatol. 2004;23(1):31–4. Epub 2004 Jan 9.

Murphey MD, Rhee JH, Lewis RB, et al. Pigmented villonodular synovitis: radiologic-pathologic correlation. Radiographics. 2008;28(5):1493–518.

Pigmented Villonodular Synovitis (PVNS): Case 16

41

41.1 Medical History

A 51-year-old female with right knee posterior mass for 10 months with numbness of the right lower leg and swelling and pain for 5 months.

41.2 Physical Examination

Palpable deep mass along the right knee with clear border, smooth, rubbery, and non-movable. No point tenderness.

41.3 Imaging Findings

41.3.1 Radiograph

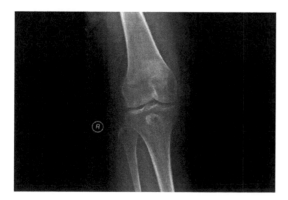

Fig. 41.1 Frontal view of the right knee

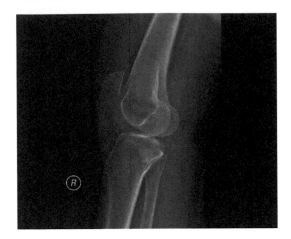

Fig. 41.2 Lateral view of the right knee

Radiographs of the right knee demonstrate focal sclerosis in the midline of the tibial plateau posteriorly with internal lucency.

41.3.2 MR Imaging

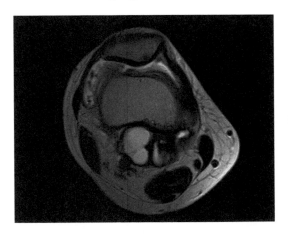

Fig. 41.3 Axial T2-weighted MR image of the right knee

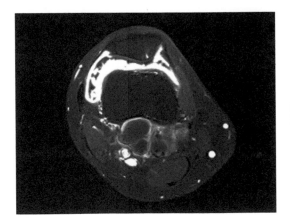

Fig. 41.4 Axial post-contrast fat-suppressed T1-weighted image of the right knee

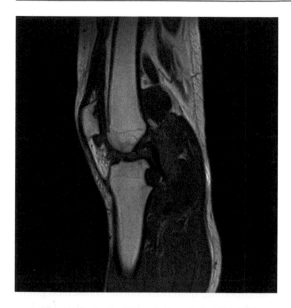

Fig. 41.5 Sagittal T1-weighted MR image of the right knee

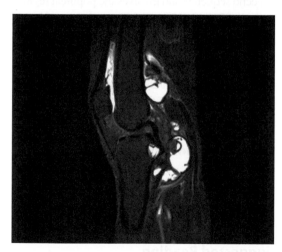

Fig. 41.6 Sagittal fat-suppressed T2-weighted MR image of the right knee

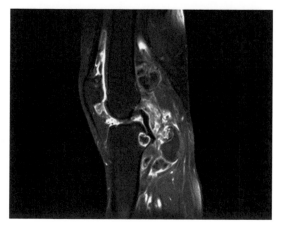

Fig. 41.7 Sagittal post-contrast fat-suppressed T1-weighted image of the right knee

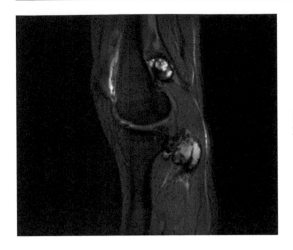

Fig. 41.8 Sagittal gradient echo MR image of the right knee

MR images of the right knee demonstrate extensive synovial hyperplasia with multiple various sized nodules. The lesions are noted surrounding the cruciate ligaments with heterogeneous enhancement. There are invasions to the distal femur and posterior tibial plateau.

41.4 Description and Discussion from Residents

Focal sclerosis with internal low density at proximal right tibia is seen on radiograph. There is a clear margin of the lesion with adjacent soft tissue swelling. Large effusion with synovial hyperplasia and nodular, heterogeneous signals at supra-patellar and popliteal region is noted on MR images. Low signal on T2-weighted images is noted, likely of hemosiderin with adjacent erosion of the cortex, not affecting the articular surface. Mild degenerative changes of the right knee are noted. Heterogeneous enhancement along the synovium is seen with avid enhancement of the proximal tibial erosion. The above findings are most consistent with pigmented villonodular synovitis (PVNS).

41.5 Analysis and Comments from Professor Cheng Xiao-Guang

Radiographs show degenerative changes of the knee with focal lesion at the proximal tibia with clear margin and increased density of the Hoffa's fat

pad. Blooming from hemosiderin is noted on gradient echo sequence and involves the popliteal region, typical of PVNS. When PVNS occurs around hip or ankle, bony erosion is usually more obvious. Tuberculosis arthropathy should be included in the differential diagnosis only when there are juxta-articular osteopenia and gradual narrowing of the joint space, not seen of the current case.

41.6 Diagnosis

Pigmented villonodular synovitis (tenosynovial giant cell tumor, diffuse type).

Suggested Reading

Cheng XG, You YH, Liu W, et al. MRI features of pigmented villonodular synovitis (PVNS). Clin Rheumatol. 2004;23(1):31–4. Epub 2004 Jan 9.
Murphey MD, Rhee JH, Lewis RB, et al. Pigmented villonodular synovitis: radiologic-pathologic correlation. Radiographics. 2008;28(5):1493–518.

Rheumatoid Arthritis: Case 17

42

42.1 Medical History

A 23-year-old female with polyarthralgia and swelling for 4 years and worsening for 9 months with morning stiffness.

42.2 Physical Examination

Limited range of motion and point tenderness at multiple joints.

42.3 Imaging Findings

42.3.1 Radiograph

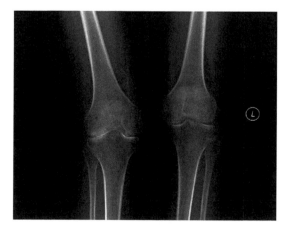

Fig. 42.1 Frontal view of both knees

© Springer Nature Singapore Pte Ltd. and Peking Union Medical College Press 2020
X. Cheng et al., *Bone Tumor Imaging*, https://doi.org/10.1007/978-981-13-9927-5_42

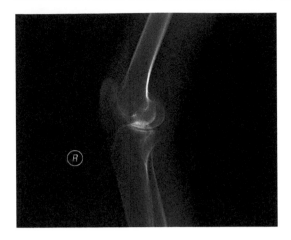

Fig. 42.2 Lateral view of the right knee

Radiographs of the knees demonstrate osteopenia of both knees with joint space loss and subchondral sclerosis.

42.4 Description and Discussion from Residents

Radiographs demonstrate osteopenia around both knees with joint space narrowing and subchondral sclerosis and soft tissue swelling, right more than left. There are also rather symmetrical both hands and feet involvements (images not provided) with marginal erosion, joint space loss, and osteopenia. There is ankylosis around the wrist with subluxation of multiple joints. Given the above imaging findings and the patient's age and clinical symptoms, this is most consistent with rheumatoid arthritis.

42.5 Analysis and Comments from Professor Cheng Xiao-Guang

Young female with multiple joints involvements and worse of the both wrists with marginal erosion, joint space loss, and osteopenia are very typical of rheumatoid arthritis.

42.6 Diagnosis

Rheumatoid arthritis.

Suggested Reading

Barile A, Arrigoni F, Bruno F, et al. Computed tomography and MR imaging in rheumatoid arthritis. Radiol Clin N Am. 2017;55(5):997–1007.

Llopis E, Kroon HM, Acosta J. Conventional radiology in rheumatoid arthritis. Radiol Clin N Am. 2017;55(5):917–41.

Sommer OJ, Kladosek A, Weiler V, et al. Rheumatoid arthritis: a practical guide to state-of-the-art imaging, image interpretation, and clinical implications. Radiographics. 2005;25(2):381–98.

Rheumatoid Arthritis: Case 18

43

43.1 Medical History

A 42-year-old female with polyarthralgia and swelling for 10 years and worsening for 7 years.

43.2 Physical Examination

Limited range of motion and point tenderness at multiple joints.

43.3 Imaging Findings

43.3.1 Radiograph

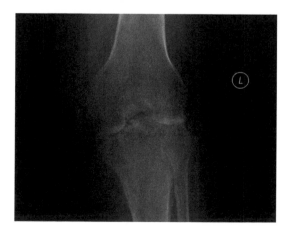

Fig. 43.1 Frontal view of the left knee

© Springer Nature Singapore Pte Ltd. and Peking Union Medical College Press 2020
X. Cheng et al., *Bone Tumor Imaging*, https://doi.org/10.1007/978-981-13-9927-5_43

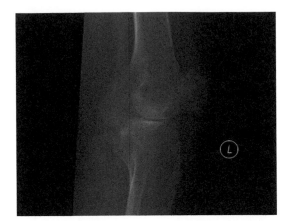

Fig. 43.2 Lateral view of the left knee

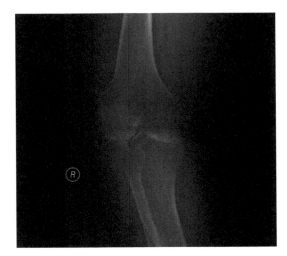

Fig. 43.3 Frontal view of the right knee

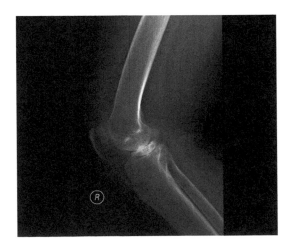

Fig. 43.4 Lateral view of the right knee

Radiographs of the knees demonstrate osteopenia of both knees with joint space loss and subchondral sclerosis.

43.4 Description and Discussion from Residents

There is marked joint space narrowing of right knee with subchondral sclerosis and soft tissue swelling. Both hands (images not provided) demonstrate multiple, symmetric marginal erosions, joint space loss with ankylosis and osteopenia. Deformity and subluxation of some joints are also noted. These typical imaging findings are consistent with rheumatoid arthritis.

43.5 Analysis and Comments from Professor Cheng Xiao-Guang

Multiple, symmetric marginal erosions of both hands and wrists with joint space narrowing or ankyloses with osteopenia and deformity or subluxation of some of the joints are typical findings

in rheumatoid arthritis. It is important to differentiate what types of joints are involved and the patterns of involvement when diagnosing arthropathy. Multiple symmetrical joints involvements with osteopenia and later joint space narrowing, ankylosis with some subluxations, and deformities are typical of rheumatoid arthritis especially of the wrists, hands, and feet.

43.6 Diagnosis

Rheumatoid arthritis.

Suggested Reading

Barile A, Arrigoni F, Bruno F, et al. Computed tomography and MR imaging in rheumatoid arthritis. Radiol Clin N Am. 2017;55(5):997–1007.

Llopis E, Kroon HM, Acosta J. Conventional radiology in rheumatoid arthritis. Radiol Clin N Am. 2017;55(5):917–41.

Sommer OJ, Kladosek A, Weiler V, et al. Rheumatoid arthritis: a practical guide to state-of-the-art imaging, image interpretation, and clinical implications. Radiographics. 2005;25(2):381–98.

Gouty Arthritis: Case 19

44

44.1 Medical History

A 60-year-old male with multiple joints alternating and recurrent redness, swelling, and pain, lasting for days and then fully resolved on its own. Now he presents with swelling of both knees with pain and squatting difficulty.

44.2 Physical Examination

Swelling and point tenderness of multiple joints with limited motion of both knees.

44.3 Imaging Findings

44.3.1 Radiograph

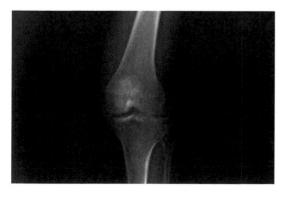

Fig. 44.1 Frontal view of the left knee

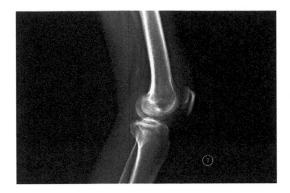

Fig. 44.2 Lateral view of the left knee

Radiographs of the left knee demonstrate soft tissue swelling and joint effusion and osteophytes formation.

44.3.2 CT Imaging

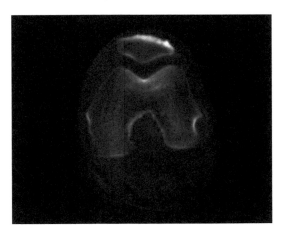

Fig. 44.3 Axial CT image of the left knee in bone window

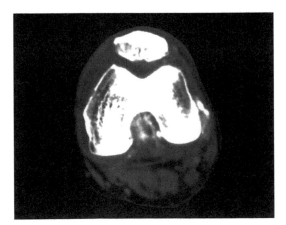

Fig. 44.4 Axial CT image of the left knee in soft tissue window

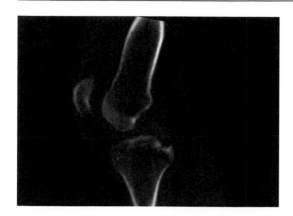

Fig. 44.5 Sagittal CT image of the left knee in bone window

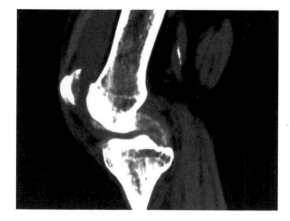

Fig. 44.6 Sagittal CT image of the left knee in soft tissue window

CT images of the left knee demonstrate large left knee effusion with synovial hyperplasia. There is osteophyte formation. Multiple calcifications are noted around cruciate and collateral ligaments.

pigmented villonodular synovitis, which would not have calcification; synovial osteochondromatosis, which usually has smooth border around the calcifications.

44.4   Description and Discussion from Residents

The patient is an older male. Radiographs demonstrate no bone destruction or erosion around the knee joint with osteophytes and soft tissue swelling. On CT scan images, there are suspicious erosion, soft tissue swelling, internal multiple calcifications, and joint effusion. The imaging findings are most suggestive of inflammatory arthropathy, and given the clinical symptoms and history, gouty arthritis is at the top of the differential diagnosis. Differential diagnosis:

44.5   Analysis and Comments from Professor Cheng Xiao-Guang

Older male patient with supra-patellar joint effusion on lateral view radiograph and no other clear abnormality; high densities noted at the intercondylar region, mainly along the ligaments on CT scan, likely of tophus and given the recurrent attacks clinically, typical of gout. Differential diagnosis includes pseudo gout which usually shows calcifications along the menisci and cartilage. Pseudo gout is relatively rare in China.

44.6   Diagnosis

Gouty arthritis.

Suggested Reading

Buckens CF, Terra MP, Maas M. Computed tomography and MR imaging in crystalline-induced Arthropathies. Radiol Clin N Am. 2017;55(5):1023–34.

Omoumi P, Zufferey P, Malghem J, et al. Imaging in gout and other crystal-related Arthropathies. Rheum Dis Clin N Am. 2016;42(4):621–44.

45.1 Medical History

A 47-year-old male with no significant clinical history and seen at outpatient clinic.

45.2 Physical Examination

No positive physical findings.

45.3 Imaging Findings

45.3.1 CT Imaging

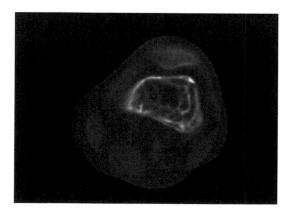

Fig. 45.1 Axial CT image of the left lower femur in bone window

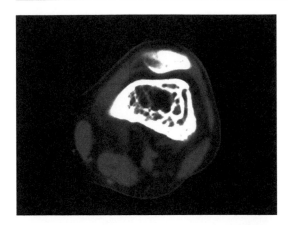

Fig. 45.2 Axial CT image of the left lower femur in soft tissue window

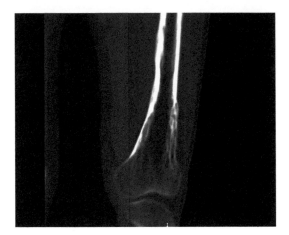

Fig. 45.3 Coronal CT image of the left lower femur in bone window

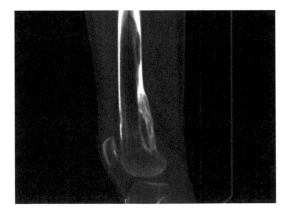

Fig. 45.4 Sagittal CT image of the left lower femur in bone window

CT images of the left knee demonstrate slightly expansile appearance of the left mid and distal femur with cortical thickening, coarsened trabeculae.

45.4 Description and Discussion from Residents

The patient is a middle-aged male. The left mid and distal femur appears to be expansile on CT scan. There is low density in the medullary cavity with coarsened trabeculae with uneven cortical thickening. There is no periosteal reaction or soft tissue mass. The above findings are most suggestive of Paget disease with fibrous dysplasia and hyperparathyroidism as differential diagnosis.

45.5 Analysis and Comments from Professor Cheng Xiao-Guang

The patient is a middle-aged male. CT images show left mid and distal femoral lesion with cortical thickening and interposed yellow marrow between the coarsened trabeculae, most suggestive of Paget disease. If there were coarsened trabeculae in one bone or multiple bones (could accompany with pain), together with elevated blood alkaline phosphatase level, diagnosis of Paget disease is confirmed. There is increased osteoclast activity in Paget disease, so therapy at control osteoclasts has good results. In contrast to fibrous dysplasia, there is normal intramedullary yellow marrow.

45.6 Diagnosis

Paget disease.

Suggested Reading

Lalam RK, Cassar-Pullicino VN, Winn N. Paget disease of bone. Semin Musculoskelet Radiol. 2016;20(3):287–99.
Smith SE, Murphey MD, Motamedi K, et al. From the archives of the AFIP. Radiologic spectrum of Paget disease of bone and its complications with pathologic correlation. Radiographics. 2002;22(5):1191–216.

Tuberculosis: Case 21

46.1 Medical History

A 7-year-old boy who was noticed with leg length discrepancy 2 years ago of longer left lower extremity and no limping.

46.2 Physical Examination

Leg length discrepancy with left lower extremity longer of 2 cm compared to the contralateral side, otherwise, no abnormality.

46.3 Imaging Findings

46.3.1 Radiograph

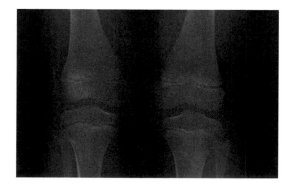

Fig. 46.1 Frontal view of the left knee

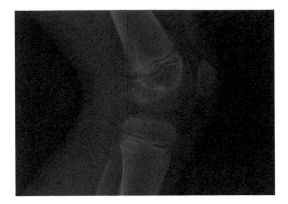

Fig. 46.2 Lateral view of the left knee

Radiographs of the left knee demonstrate distal left femoral epiphyseal lytic lesion with peripheral sclerosis and internal higher densities.

46.3.2 CT Imaging

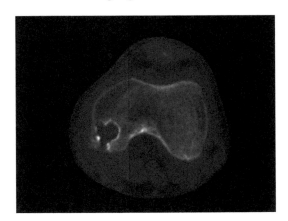

Fig. 46.3 Axial CT image of the left knee in bone window

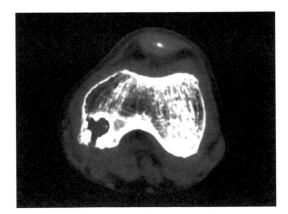

Fig. 46.4 Axial CT image of the left knee in soft tissue window

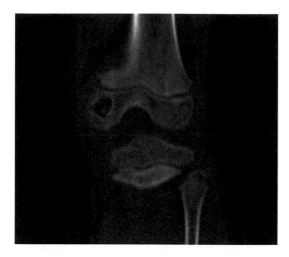

Fig. 46.5 Coronal CT image of the left knee in bone window

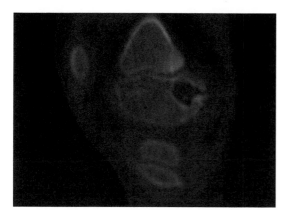

Fig. 46.6 Sagittal CT image of the left knee in bone window

CT images of the left knee demonstrate destructive lesion at the distal left femoral epiphysis with clear border and internal high densities.

46.3.3 MR Imaging

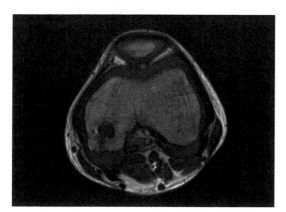

Fig. 46.7 Axial T1-weighted MR image of the left knee

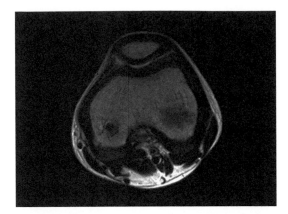

Fig. 46.8 Axial T2-weighted MR image of the left knee

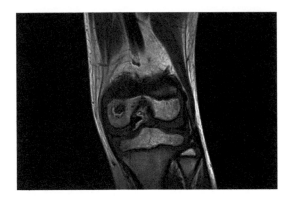

Fig. 46.9 Coronal T1-weighted MR image of the left knee

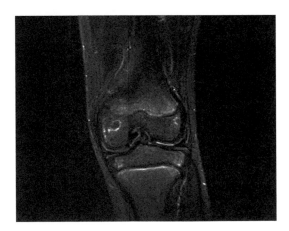

Fig. 46.10 Coronal fat-suppressed T2-weighted MR image of the left knee

MR images of the right knee demonstrate the semicircular lesion with a 0.9 cm diameter. There is slightly irregular border posteriorly with internal iso T1 and low T2 signals. On the fat-suppressed sequence, there is a peripheral circular high signal without much surrounding edema.

46.4 Description and Discussion from Residents

The patient is a young child. Radiographs demonstrate left distal femoral epiphyseal semicircular lytic lesion with peripheral sclerosis. On CT scan images, the peripheral sclerosis is obvious with internal high densities, hard to differentiate if that is chondroid matrix or fragments. There is a posterior cortical break. No obvious inflammation is noted around the joint. The imaging findings are most suggestive of tuberculosis or chondroblastoma. On MR images, there is no chondroid matrix in the lesion, some fatty tissues are noted, and there is no marrow edema around the lesion with posterior cortical break; tuberculosis is at the top of the diagnosis.

46.5 Analysis and Comments from Professor Cheng Xiao-Guang

There is a distal femoral epiphyseal destructive lesion with clear border and peripheral sclerosis; chondroblastoma can be considered. CT images demonstrate posterior cortical break, suggesting a sinus track, not typical of chondroblastoma. There is not much adjacent soft tissue inflammation, not typical of tuberculosis or chondroblastoma. The lesion is without much enhancement. On the MR images, there is a fat signal at the peripheral of the lesion with mild adjacent edema. The combination of imaging findings is most suggestive of tuberculosis.

46.6 Diagnosis

Tuberculosis.

Suggested Reading

De Backer AI, Mortelé KJ, Vanhoenacker FM, et al. Imaging of extraspinal musculoskeletal tuberculosis. Eur J Radiol. 2006;57(1):119–30.

Prasad A, Manchanda S, Sachdev N, et al. Imaging features of pediatric musculoskeletal tuberculosis. Pediatr Radiol. 2012;42(10):1235–49.

Giant Cell Tumor of Bone: Case 22

47

47.1 Medical History

A 21-year-old male with left knee twisting injury 7 months ago complains of joint swelling and pain. The pain resolved after rest but swelling persists.

47.2 Physical Examination

Swelling around the lateral and proximal aspect of left lower leg, hard, and with point tenderness.

47.3 Imaging Findings

47.3.1 Radiograph

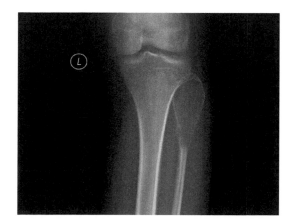

Fig. 47.1 Frontal view of the left proximal fibula

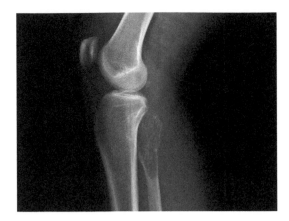

Fig. 47.2 Lateral view of the left proximal fibula

Radiographs of the left proximal fibula demon-strate expansile bone destruction without perios-teal reaction.

47.3.2 CT Imaging

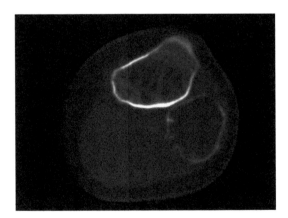

Fig. 47.3 Axial CT image of the left proximal fibula in bone window

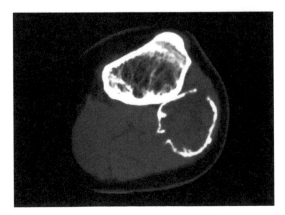

Fig. 47.4 Axial CT image of the left proximal fibula in soft tissue window

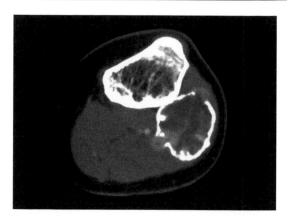

Fig. 47.5 Axial post-contrast CT image of the left proximal fibula in soft tissue window

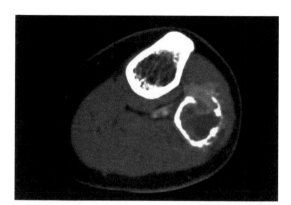

Fig. 47.6 Axial post-contrast CT image of the left proximal fibula in soft tissue window

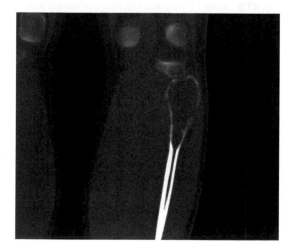

Fig. 47.7 Coronal CT image of the left proximal fibula in bone window

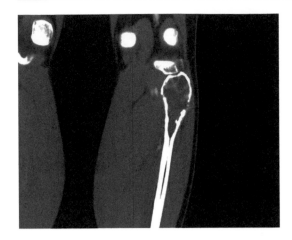

Fig. 47.8 Coronal post-contrast CT image of the left proximal fibula in soft tissue window

CT images of the left proximal fibula demonstrate an expansile lytic lesion with focal cortical break and internal cystic changes. There is enhancement of the solid component.

47.3.3 MR Imaging

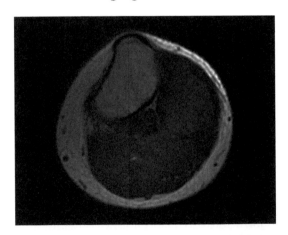

Fig. 47.9 Axial T1-weighted MR image of the left proximal fibula

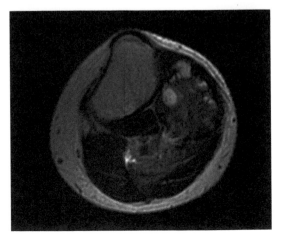

Fig. 47.10 Axial T2-weighted MR image of the left proximal fibula

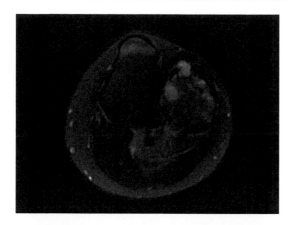

Fig. 47.11 Axial fat-suppressed T2-weighted MR image of the left proximal fibula

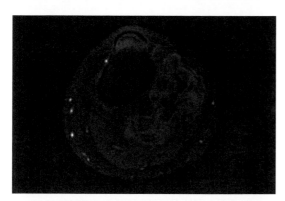

Fig. 47.12 Axial post-contrast fat-suppressed T1-weighted MR image of the left proximal fibula

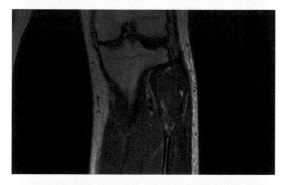

Fig. 47.13 Coronal T1-weighted MR image of the left proximal fibula

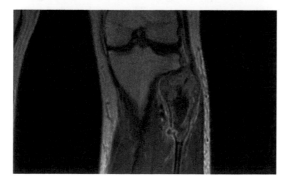

Fig. 47.14 Coronal post-contrast T1-weigthted MR image of the left proximal fibula

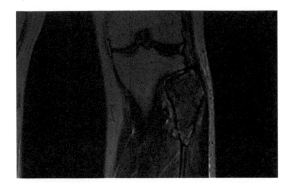

Fig. 47.15 Coronal T2-weighted MR image of the left proximal fibula

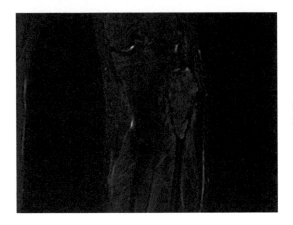

Fig. 47.16 Coronal fat-suppressed T2-weighted MR image of the left proximal fibula

MR images of the left proximal fibula demonstrate mixed T1 and T2 signals of the lesion, with majority of low signal. There is peripheral enhancement.

47.4 Description and Discussion from Residents

The patient is a young male. Radiographs demonstrate left proximal fibular expansile lytic lesion with cortical break and no significant periosteal reaction, nor soft tissue swelling. There is clear bone destruction on CT scan with internal heterogeneous densities and cystic changes. The solid component is noted to extend beyond the cortical break with enhancement, most suggestive of giant cell tumor of bone. There is high T1 signal within the lesion, suggestive of hemor-

rhage on MR images, and there is low T2 signal with heterogeneous enhancement, again most suggestive of giant cell tumor of bone.

47.5 Analysis and Comments from Professor Cheng Xiao-Guang

The patient is a young male. Radiographs demonstrate expansile lytic lesion at the left proximal fibula with pathological fracture and no significant periosteal reaction. There are heterogeneous densities within the lesion on CT scan without calcification and with cortical break and enhancement of the solid component of the lesion. Majority of the lesion demonstrates low T1 and T2 signals with heterogeneous enhancement, most suggestive of giant cell tumor of bone.

47.6 Diagnosis

Giant cell tumor of bone.

Suggested Reading

Chakarun CJ, Forrester DM, Gottsegen CJ, et al. Giant cell tumor of bone: review, mimics, and new developments in treatment. Radiographics. 2013;33(1):197–211.

Denison GL, Workman TL. General case of the day. Benign giant cell tumor with extension through the fibular head into the adjacent soft tissue. Radiographics. 1997;17(2):545–7.

Murphey MD, Nomikos GC, Flemming DJ, et al. From the archives of AFIP. Imaging of giant cell tumor and giant cell reparative granuloma of bone: radiologic-pathologic correlation. Radiographics. 2001;21(5):1283–309.

48.1 Medical History

A 50-year-old female with knee pain seen at out-patient clinic.

48.2 Physical Examination

Tenderness.

48.3 Imaging Findings

48.3.1 Radiograph

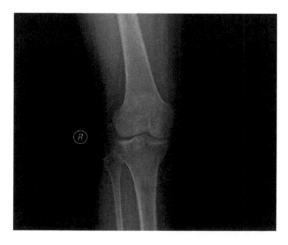

Fig. 48.1 Frontal view of the right knee

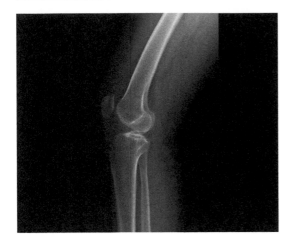

Fig. 48.2 Lateral view of the right knee

Radiographs of the right knee demonstrate low density lesions at the tibial plateau and femoral condyle with peripheral sclerosis.

48.3.2 CT Imaging

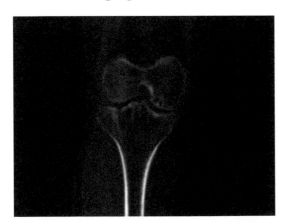

Fig. 48.3 Coronal CT scan of the right knee in bone window

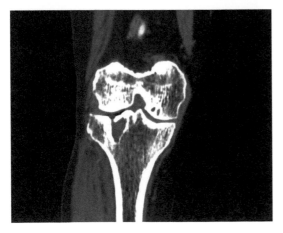

Fig. 48.4 Coronal post-contrast CT scan of the right knee in soft tissue window

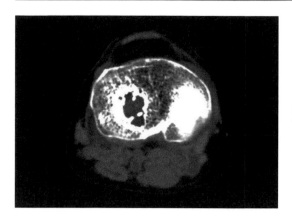

Fig. 48.5 Axial CT scan of the right knee in soft tissue window

CT images of the right knee demonstrate the cystic lesions at the medial femoral condyle and lateral tibial plateau with peripheral sclerosis. Vacuum phenomenon is seen at the lateral compartment. The cysts are communicating with the joint.

48.4 Description and Discussion from Residents

The patient is an older female. There are degenerative changes of the knee with low densities at the femoral condyle and tibial plateau with peripheral sclerosis on radiographs. The cystic changes are communicating with the joint with internal high densities on CT scan and consistent with subchondral cysts (geode).

48.5 Analysis and Comments from Professor Cheng Xiao-Guang

The patient is an older female. Radiographs demonstrate degenerative changes of the knee with tibial plateau cystic lesion with peripheral sclero-sis and similar changes at the femoral condyle. On the CT scan, the lesions are well circumscribed and communicating with the joint. These lesions are consistent with subchondral cysts, without need to differentiate from benign neoplasm. First, the lesion is just below the articular surface, and second, neoplastic lesion is usually more expansile from internal tension. The current case shows collapse of the tibial plateau, indicating low internal tension.

48.6 Diagnosis

Subchondral cyst.

Suggested Reading

Jacobson JA, Girish G, Jiang Y, et al. Radiographic evaluation of arthritis: degenerative joint disease and variations. Radiology. 2008;248(3):737–47.
Stacy GS, Peabody TD, Dixon LB. Mimics on radiography of giant cell tumor of bone. AJR Am J Roentgenol. 2003;181(6):1583–9.

49.1 Medical History

A 56-year-old female with right knee pain seen at outpatient clinic.

49.2 Physical Examination

Tenderness.

49.3 Imaging Findings

49.3.1 Radiograph

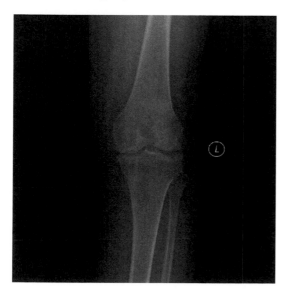

Fig. 49.1 Frontal view of the left knee

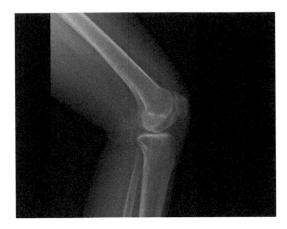

Fig. 49.2 Lateral view of the left knee

Radiographs of the left knee demonstrate irregular low-density area at the proximal tibial plateau with peripheral sclerosis.

49.3.2 CT Imaging

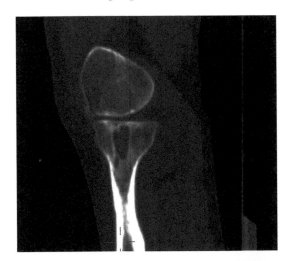

Fig. 49.3 Sagittal CT scan of the left knee in bone window

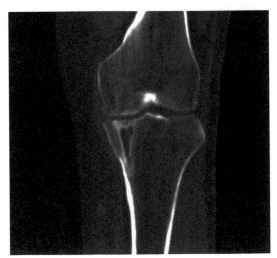

Fig. 49.4 Coronal CT scan of the left knee in bone window

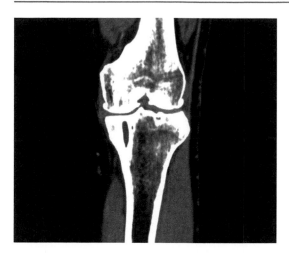

Fig. 49.5 Coronal CT scan of the left knee in soft tissue window

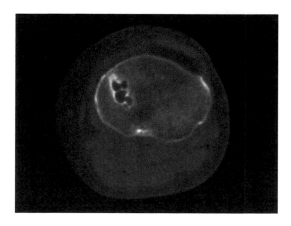

Fig. 49.6 Axial CT scan of the left knee in bone window

CT images of the left knee demonstrate similar findings as on radiograph. There is communication of the lesion with the joint.

49.4 Description and Discussion from Residents

The patient is an older female. There is tibial plateau lesion with similar lesion at the medial femoral condyle with peripheral sclerosis on radiographs. CT scan images better depict the lesions and show the communication with the joint, most consistent with subchondral cyst (geode).

49.5 Analysis and Comments from Professor Cheng Xiao-Guang

The patient is an older female. Radiographs demonstrate degenerative changes of the knee with tibial plateau cystic lesion with peripheral sclerosis. CT images better demonstrate the peripheral sclerosis and consistent with subchondral cyst. There are many causes for development of subchondral cystic changes. The most common cause is osteoarthritis, just as in the current case. A differential diagnosis is juxta-articular bone cyst, which is not related to joint pathology and not necessarily need to communicate with the joint.

49.6   Diagnosis

Subchondral cyst.

Suggested Reading

Jacobson JA, Girish G, Jiang Y, et al. Radiographic evaluation of arthritis: degenerative joint disease and variations. Radiology. 2008;248(3):737–47.

Stacy GS, Peabody TD, Dixon LB. Mimics on radiography of giant cell tumor of bone. AJR Am J Roentgenol. 2003;181(6):1583–9.

Extraskeletal Myxoid Chondrosarcoma: Case 25

50

50.1 Medical History

A 75-year-old male with enlarging mass at the back of the left thigh for 6 months.

50.2 Physical Examination

Palpable mass at posterior thigh without point tenderness and normal range of motion of the joint.

50.3 Imaging Findings

50.3.1 Radiograph

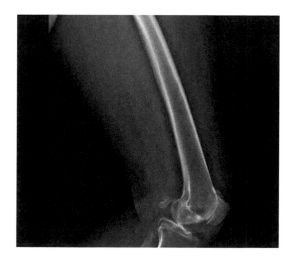

Fig. 50.1 Lateral view of the left femur

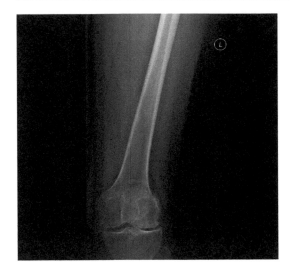

Fig. 50.2 Frontal view of the left femur

Radiographs of the left femur demonstrate soft tissue prominence at the mid left thigh posteriorly.

50.3.2 CT Imaging

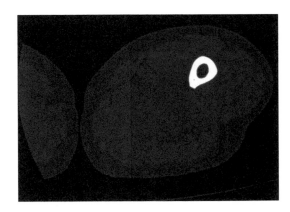

Fig. 50.3 Axial CT scan of the left mid femur in bone window

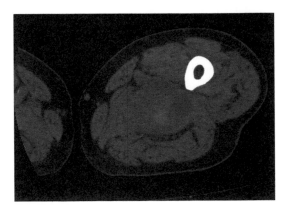

Fig. 50.4 Axial CT scan of the left mid femur in soft tissue window

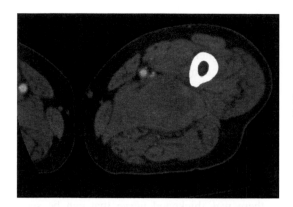

Fig. 50.5 Axial post-contrast CT scan of the left mid femur in soft tissue window

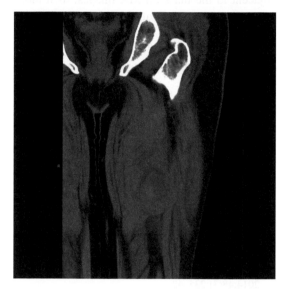

Fig. 50.6 Coronal CT scan of the left mid femur in soft tissue window

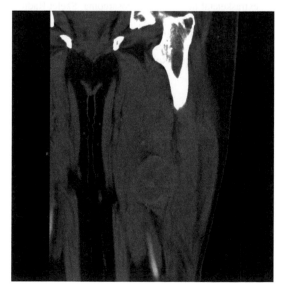

Fig. 50.7 Coronal post-contrast CT scan of the left mid femur in soft tissue window

CT images of the left mid femur demonstrate a soft tissue mass along the mid left thigh in the medial and posterior aspect, without clear border. There is internal high-density area. Peripheral enhancement is seen. No invasion of the underlying femur is noted.

50.4 Description and Discussion from Residents

Ill-defined soft tissue mass is noted on radiograph at the mid left thigh without invasion to the femur or periosteal reaction. Internal high densities are noted on CT scan, which could represent hemorrhage. Heterogeneous enhancement is seen at peripheral and center of the mass. There are internal septations and necrosis without destructive changes of the adjacent femur. The above findings favor malignant process.

50.5 Analysis and Comments from Professor Cheng Xiao-Guang

The patient is an older male. Radiographs demonstrate soft tissue mass at mid left thigh with relatively high density. CT scan images demonstrate heterogeneous low density of the lesion without clear border. There are patchy high densities, likely of hemorrhage. The surrounding fat appears preserved. Focal avid enhancements are noted. When evaluating a soft tissue tumor on imaging, first, the location is important. The deeper the mass is, the more likely it is malignant. If the mass is adjacent to a neurovascular bundle, then nerve sheath tumor is likely. Second, the internal density of the lesion is important, such as presence of calcification or fat. The current case, given patient's age, is most likely a malignant lesion. Liposarcoma and malignant fibrous histiocytoma are in the differential diagnosis. Additionally, the current lesion is oval with preserved fat plane and adjacent to neurovascular bundle, so nerve sheath tumor cannot be excluded. If there was thickened nerve that can be seen adjacent to the mass on MR images, then more suggestive of nerve sheath tumor.

50.6 Diagnosis

Extraskeletal myxoid chondrosarcoma, given positive S100 protein, should be differentiated from low-grade malignant peripheral nerve sheath tumor.

Suggested Reading

Kapoor N, Shinagare AB, Jagannathan JP, et al. Clinical and radiologic features of extraskeletal myxoid chondrosarcoma including initial presentation, local recurrence, and metastases. Radiol Oncol. 2014;48(3):235–42.

Tateishi U, Hasegawa T, Nojima T, et al. MRI features of extraskeletal myxoid chondrosarcoma. Skelet Radiol. 2006;35(1):27–33.

Zhang L, Wang R, Xu R, et al. Extraskeletal myxoid chondrosarcoma: a comparative study of imaging and pathology. Biomed Res Int. 2018;2018:9684268.

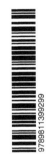

9789811399299